Workbook for

Elsevier's Veterinary Assisting Textbook

Workbook for

Elsevier's Veterinary Assisting Textbook

Margi Sirois, EdD, MS, RVT, LAT
Ashworth College
Norcross, Georgia

With 106 figures

ELSEVIER

ELSEVIER

3251 Riverport Lane
St. Louis, Missouri 63043

WORKBOOK FOR ELSEVIER'S VETERINARY ASSISTING TEXTBOOK,
SECOND EDITION   ISBN: 978-0-323-37710-2

Notices

Knowledge and best practice in this field are constantly changing. As new research and experience broaden our understanding, changes in research methods, professional practices, or medical treatment may become necessary.

Practitioners and researchers must always rely on their own experience and knowledge in evaluating and using any information, methods, compounds, or experiments described herein. In using such information or methods they should be mindful of their own safety and the safety of others, including parties for whom they have a professional responsibility.

With respect to any drug or pharmaceutical products identified, readers are advised to check the most current information provided (i) on procedures featured or (ii) by the manufacturer of each product to be administered, to verify the recommended dose or formula, the method and duration of administration, and contraindications. It is the responsibility of practitioners, relying on their own experience and knowledge of their patients, to make diagnoses, to determine dosages and the best treatment for each individual patient, and to take all appropriate safety precautions.

To the fullest extent of the law, neither the Publisher nor the authors, contributors, or editors, assume any liability for any injury and/or damage to persons or property as a matter of products liability, negligence or otherwise, or from any use or operation of any methods, products, instructions, or ideas contained in the material herein.

Previous edition copyrighted 2013.

Content Strategist: Brandi Graham
Senior Content Development Specialist: Diane Chatman
Publishing Services Manager: Hemamalini Rajendrababu
Senior Project Manager: Beula Christopher
Designer: Margaret Reid

Working together
to grow libraries in
developing countries

www.elsevier.com • www.bookaid.org

Printed in United States of America

Last digit is the print number: 9   8   7   6   5   4   3   2   1

Preface

This workbook is intended to accompany *Elsevier's Veterinary Assisting Textbook,* 2nd edition. Each chapter in the workbook relates to a corresponding chapter in the textbook and stresses the essential information of the chapter through the use of definitions, short essays (comprehension), photo quizzes, matching, completion, true and false, multiple choice questions, word searches, and crossword puzzles.

Learning objectives are included at the beginning of each chapter to help you focus on the material and concepts that you are expected to learn and how this is to be applied in the veterinary clinical setting.

The following suggestions will help you use this workbook to identify strengths and weaknesses.

1. Review the contents of each chapter before you attempt to do the exercise. Do not treat the questions individually and then refer to the text for the correct answer. Deal with the chapter's subject matter as a whole, because many of the questions are interrelated.

This is a learning exercise meant to help you learn the material presented in the textbook, not an examination for grades.

2. Remember that the same subject matter may be repeated in different question forms in each chapter or other chapters, because the material overlaps. The subjects of the questions are not in the same order as they appear in the textbook.

3. Read each question and study each illustration carefully before answering. You may know the answer or you may arrive at the correct answer by knowing which answers are incorrect.

4. This workbook is designed so that the pages can be easily removed, submitted if required, and placed in your notebook with the corresponding lecture notes.

The answers to all the exercises appear in the *Instructor Resources for Elsevier's Veterinary Assisting Textbook,* 2nd edition, on the Evolve website.

Contents

1 Overview of the Veterinary Profession

LEARNING OBJECTIVES

After reviewing this chapter, the reader will be able to:

- Describe educational requirements of veterinary team members.
- Define appropriate nomenclature describing veterinary personnel.
- Identify the duties of the members of the veterinary health care team.
- Recognize professional organizations supporting veterinary medicine.
- Discuss ethical issues and guidelines relevant to the veterinary profession.
- List and describe general categories of laws relevant to the veterinary profession.
- Define laws protecting veterinary employees against physical injury, sexual harassment, and discrimination.
- Explain laws relating to ensuring quality veterinary service.

TRUE OR FALSE

1. _____ The employing veterinarian has the ultimate responsibility for using a veterinary assistant in an appropriate and ethical manner, consistent with state and federal law.

2. _____ For a reasonable annual fee, membership in the Veterinary Support Personnel Network allows assistants to participate in online continuing education, live chats, and surveys.

3. _____ A society has bylaws, leaders, and committees designed to oversee technician specialty certification.

4. _____ Veterinary assistants are not licensed, and in most states their role is not clearly defined.

5. _____ Veterinary assistants should excel at physical restraint, animal grooming, and inventory control.

6. _____ The area described as the "front" of a veterinary practice is the area used for lab work.

7. _____ Veterinary technicians who maintain their certification, registration, or license after passing the VTNE are referred to as *credentialed veterinary technicians.*

8. _____ The veterinary team member most responsible for prescribing medication is the veterinary technician.

9. _____ Team efficiency improves and benchmark standards are achieved when veterinary practice management is doctor centered.

10. _____ One way to create a comfortable reception area is to provide clients with cozy, close seating; floor plants for ambiance; and many magazines.

FILL IN THE BLANK

1. The majority of veterinarians are involved in _____ practices.

2. Veterinarians who have special expertise in one aspect of medicine may offer services in a _____ practice.

3. Most veterinary hospital staff members wear _____ or laboratory jackets.

4. Valuable items on display in the retail area should be placed behind the _____ area.

5. Duties of the _____ usually includes restraining, feeding, and exercising patients; cleaning the hospital and boarding premises; and performing other clinical support tasks.

6. The back of the practice generally includes the radiology, surgery, and _____ areas.

7. The middle portion of a veterinary practice contains _____, _____, and _____ areas.

8. When someone does something unethical, it is not necessarily considered _____.

9. The laws that govern the veterinary profession are written in the _____.

10. _____ is an online tool offering region-specific cost-of-living and salary information for veterinary personnel.

SHORT ANSWER

1. Define the *human-animal bond*.

   _____

2. To avoid injury, how best is animal restraint managed?

   _____

   _____

3. What is the purpose of a dosimetry badge?

   _____

4. The National Fire Protection Association (NFPA) suggests that you do not attempt to fight a fire under what conditions?

   _____

   _____

   _____

5. According to common law practice, what must a plaintiff prove in a malpractice or professional negligence suit?

   _____

   _____

6. What types of materials may be considered medical waste?

   _____

7. What is the definition of *ethics*?

   _____

   _____

8. What is the purpose of the Occupational Safety and Health Administration (OSHA)?

   _____

9. Describe the one-handed method for recapping a needle.

   _____

   _____

10. What is the purpose of the Hazardous Materials Plan?

   _____

LISTS

1. List seven possible members of the veterinary team:

    1. _____

    2. _____

    3. _____

    4. _____

    5. _____

    6. _____

    7. _____

2. List nine responsibilities of a veterinary assistant:

    1. _____

    2. _____

    3. _____

    4. _____

    5. _____

    6. _____

    7. _____

    8. _____

    9. _____

3. List seven areas or zones in a veterinary practice:

    1. _____

    2. _____

    3. _____

    4. _____

    5. _____

    6. _____

    7. _____

4. List three key safety steps for operating machinery and moving parts of equipment:

    1. _____

    2. _____

    3. _____

5. List the laws that ensure the quality of veterinary services:

    1. _____

    2. _____

    3. _____

6. List the laws that provide a safe business environment:

   1. _____

   2. _____

   3. _____

7. List the seven areas of safety in the workplace that OSHA addresses:

   1. _____

   2. _____

   3. _____

   4. _____

   5. _____

   6. _____

   7. _____

8. List the two hazards to be concerned about during bathing and dipping procedures:

   1. _____

   2. _____

9. List the five zoonotic hazards encountered in veterinary practice:

   1. _____

   2. _____

   3. _____

   4. _____

   5. _____

10. List the steps for handling ethylene oxide:

    1. _____

    2. _____

    3. _____

    4. _____

    5. _____

    6. _____

    7. _____

11. List the types of veterinary practices:

    1. _____

    2. _____

    3. _____

    4. _____

    5. _____

MATCHING

Match the group with its purpose.

1. _____ Academy

2. _____ NAVTA

3. _____ Society

A. Fosters high standards of veterinary care and promotes the veterinary health care team

B. Association of professionals with common interests

C. Specialty group involved in credentialing of individuals

Match the team member with the description.

1. _____ Veterinary Assistant

2. _____ Veterinary Technician

3. _____ Veterinary Technologist

4. _____ Veterinary Technician Specialist

5. _____ Veterinarian

A. A person who has graduated from a 2-year AVMA-accredited program

B. A person who has graduated from a 4-year CVTEA-accredited program

C. A person with the training of a clinical aide

D. A person who has graduated from a 4-year AVMA-accredited program receiving a Doctor of Veterinary Medicine degree

E. Credentialed technician who meets requirements established by an academy

FILL IN THE CHART

Select the appropriate personal protective equipment (PPE) required for each of the following procedures.

Personal Protective Equipment

1. latex gloves
2. surgical mask
3. leather gloves
4. personal hearing protection
5. scavenger unit
6. ventilation fan
7. impact-resistant goggles
8. lead-lined apron, thyroid collar, gloves, lead-impregnated glasses
9. protective apron
10. wash hands following the procedure with disinfectant soap

Procedure	PPE Required
Holding a stray, wild, or unvaccinated animal	
Handling a fractious animal	
Cleaning kennel cages	
Bathing and dipping	
Handling specimens	
Handling animals infectious to humans	
Mixing, transferring, agitating, or transporting chemicals	
Administering anesthesia	
Exposing radiographs	
Filling anesthesia machine vaporizer	
Changing soda lime in anesthesia lines	
Connecting and disconnecting anesthesia tanks	

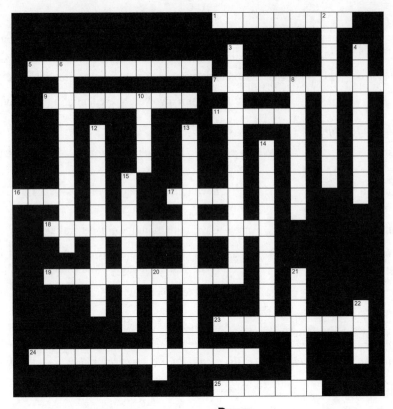

Across

1. A ___ badge measures scatter radiation
5. A veterinary __ has graduated from a 4-year AVMA-accredited program
7. Negligence that causes injury to the patient
9. A veterinary __ has graduated from a 2-year AVMA-accredited program
11. The system of moral principles that determines appropriate behavior and actions
16. Act designed to provide a safe workplace for everyone working in any business affecting commerce
17. Acronym for the national organization that is the voice of veterinary technicians
18. Keeps the patients clean and alerts the team of any changes in patient status
19. Person responsible for overseeing the front office staff as well as training receptionists to excel at customer service and public relations
23. Personal ___ equipment includes gloves, masks, and goggles
24. The special, healthy relationship between people and their pets
25. The person who bathes, brushes, and clips animals

Down

2. The ___ Law requires that you be informed about all chemicals to which you may be exposed while doing your job
3. Team member who handles client and personnel issues, supervises training sessions for team members, and holds team members accountable for their actions
4. Veterinary __ is the science and art of providing professional support service to veterinarians
6. A __ veterinary technician is a person who has graduated from an AVMA-accredited program, passed the VTNE, and maintains certification, registration, or licensure in the state in which he or she lives
8. A veterinary __ is a person who has the training of a clinical aide; who excels at physical restraint, basic laboratory skills, patient care, and client relations; and who assists veterinary technicians and veterinarians
10. Acronym for the committee that accredits veterinary technician programs
12. A person with a DVM degree
13. A ___ practice specializes in treating family pets
14. The "face" of the veterinary practice
15. Failure to exercise the necessary legal obligation of skill and diligence in treating a patient
20. Establishes its own bylaws; leaders; and application, testing, and credentialing committees, and tests only those candidates who meet specific requirements
21. The Veterinary __ Act is the law governing veterinary medicine in a state
22. The veterinary __ consists of a veterinarian, veterinary technician, assistants, receptionists, and hospital managers

2 Office Procedures and Client Relations

LEARNING OBJECTIVES

After reviewing this chapter, the reader will be able to:

- Describe the importance of informed consent.
- Clarify admitting and discharge instructions.
- Identify effective and professional discharge sheets.
- Define and educate clients regarding Pet Health Insurance.
- Identify a completed medical record.
- Identify and use POMR and SOAP record formats.
- Identify methods used to accurately and efficiently maintain inventory.
- Develop effective phone techniques.
- Identify techniques for handling multiple phone lines.
- Describe methods to greet clients effectively.
- Differentiate forms used in the veterinary practice.

FILL IN THE BLANK

1. Teamwork helps facilitate _____ _____ for clients and employees.

2. The quality of voice is a combination of _____, _____, _____ and _____.

3. The stock level that an item reaches before it is reordered is referred to as the _____.

4. The ultimate goal of inventory costs is that they should total _____% to _____% of the overall income of the practice.

5. Shrinkage is defined as _____.

6. In order to put _____ at ease, a warm welcome from and accessibility of team members is a must.

7. The client's experience starts with the first _____ and ends when the practice has _____ up after the visit.

8. If the client has to call the practice to receive test results, this can leave a _____ impression.

9. The receptionist should answer the phone within _____ rings.

10. Information can be misinterpreted, especially over the phone; a pet's condition must never be _____ over the phone!

11. A recommendation given to a client over the phone must be _____ in the medical record.

12. Appointment schedules should be developed to _____ production while _____ client wait time.

13. _____ _____ are issued by the U.S. Department of Agriculture and by the state and may be required for interstate and international travel.

14. A valid _____ relationship must exist for a veterinarian to dispense prescription products.

15. When the receptionist details the entire _____ for the client, it shows the total charges for the visit.

16. Accounts receivable totals should never exceed _____% to _____% of the total gross revenue amount of the practice.

17. To facilitate prosecution of "bad check" writers, a _____ number must be written on the check.

18. A collections agency's report can remain on a client's credit report for _____ years.

19. On discharge from the hospital, patients must be released with _____ instructions.

20. Discharge instructions should be given and payment should be made **before** or **after** (circle one) the pet is brought to the client.

21. The increased use of pet _____ is expected to decrease the number of euthanasia procedures performed each year because of the cost of medical care.

22. Indemnity insurance offers _____ for treatment of injured and sick pets.

23. A _____ is defined as the amount an owner pays monthly or annually to maintain an insurance policy for a pet.

24. A _____ is the amount an owner must pay before the insurance company will offer compensation.

25. A co-pay is the _____ that the owner is responsible for after the deductible has been met.

26. Insurance may be denied because of a _____ condition—an abnormality transmitted by genes from parent to offspring.

27. Backing up documents _____ prevents thieves from stealing the most current copy of data from the practice if they are removing all the computer equipment or if a fire or natural disaster occurs.

28. **True** or **False** (circle one): It is acceptable for a veterinary assistant to sign the rabies certificate as long as the veterinarian is present.

29. Costs associated with expired medications, ordering, shipping, insurance, and taxes are _____ costs.

30. Surgical patients must be examined within _____ hours prior to receiving anesthesia.

31. Small animals flying in the United States may require an _____.

32. **True** or **False** (circle one): Blanket consent forms are recommended in the practice of veterinary medicine.

33. A medical record is a legal document that must be maintained for _____ years if the client has not returned to the practice.

34. If computerized records are used, _____ accuracy is necessary for all data entry; incorrectly entered computer records may never be retrieved.

35. The most common error made is not documenting the communication with the owner regarding the _____ of the patient.

36. A goal for the inventory manager is to not exceed the average shelf life of an item, which is _____ months.

37. The number of times inventory turns over in a practice within a specified time is referred to as _____.

38. When a current client-patient-veterinarian relationship exists, a _____ product can be sold.

39. _____ is one of the largest expenses in the practice.

40. A product markup must be at least _____% in order for the practice to break even.

41. Practices may add a _____ fee as well as a minimum prescription charge.

42. Computers function optimally for only _____ to _____ years and then need to be replaced.

43. Clients draw preliminary conclusions within the first _____ to _____ minutes of entering the building.

44. After a puppy or kitten examination, clients should be sent home with written material about _____

and _____.

SHORT ANSWER

1. Explain why an orthopedic appointment is given more time than a yearly vaccination appointment.

_____

_____

_____

_____

2. Explain how positive employee body language can increase compliance.

_____

_____

_____

_____

3. Describe how lack of eye contact can create a negative impression for the client.

_____

_____

_____

_____

4. How do reminder calls help the practice and the clients?

_____

_____

_____

_____

5. How can dropping a pet off at the clinic be of great service to the client?

_____

_____

_____

_____

6. How can you greet a client if you are on the phone or already helping another client?

_____

_____

_____

_____

7. Explain why most new patient/client forms have to include a phone number and driver's license number.

_____

_____

_____

_____

8. Explain what a blanket consent form is and why it isn't the best form to use.

_____

_____

_____

_____

9. List the information that must be included on a rabies certificate.

Owner Information   **Patient Information**   **Veterinary Information**

_____   _____   _____

_____   _____   _____

_____   _____

                                   _____

                                   _____

10. List the six stages of grief.

_____

_____

_____

_____

11. Describe ways in which the veterinary staff members can assist bereaved pet owners.

_____

_____

_____

_____

12. List some of the things the veterinary assistant can educate clients about during the office visit.

_____

_____

_____

_____

13. If admitting a patient, the client needs to sign some forms; what would these most likely be?

_____

_____

_____

_____

14. List ways in which the veterinary staff members can achieve closure with a bereaved pet owner.

_____

_____

_____

_____

15. Phone etiquette involves several elements. Explain how the tone of the person answering the call can create a positive or a negative impression.

_____

_____

_____

_____

16. What effects can the loss of a patient have on the staff?

_____

_____

_____

_____

17. Explain why medical records are legal documents and how they should be written to maintain the document.

_____

_____

_____

_____

18. If a clinic uses paperless medical records, why is it important that all documentation be done in a timely manner?

_____

_____

_____

_____

19. What do the acronyms *POMR* and *SOAP* stand for with regard to medical records?

_____

_____

_____

_____

20. What commonly overlooked errors and incomplete medical records can be caught by diligent team members?

_____

_____

_____

_____

21. What are SOPs, and why are they so useful in the veterinary practice?

_____

_____

_____

_____

22. Describe the qualities an inventory manager should have.

_____

_____

_____

_____

23. What are the costs associated with ordering a product for the clinic?

_____

_____

_____

_____

24. Explain how a practice would "mark up" a product.

_____

_____

_____

_____

25. Give three examples of products that can be sold by a veterinarian only when the relationship exists with the client and patient.

_____

_____

_____

26. List what must be on a prescription label before the prescribed medication leaves the practice.

_____

_____

_____

_____

27. Rewrite this direction so it is more concise: "Give 1 capsule every 8 hours for 1 week."

_____

_____

28. Explain how the human-animal bond has evolved over time and why this concept is important for the veterinary team to understand.

_____

_____

_____

_____

29. Who owns the medical records of patients? If records are needed by another practitioner, describe the transfer process.

_____

_____

30. How can computers benefit a veterinary practice?

_____

_____

_____

_____

31. How do team members learn how to use management software?

_____

_____

32. Describe what makes up voice quality and one way to practice good phone etiquette.

_____

_____

33. List the elements a patient history should contain.

_____

_____

34. The patient's bill states "DHLPP injection." What would be a better way to describe this service on the invoice?

_____

_____

35. Explain the use of R/I and R/O and how they apply to SOAP.

_____

_____

_____

_____

_____

_____

WORD SEARCH

Fill in the blanks, and then find the words in the word search below.

1. An animal owner who pays for services and goods is a _____.

2. All personnel in a veterinary practice are referred to as the _____.

3. A piece of office equipment that manipulates data according to a set of instructions is a _____.

4. An animal in a veterinary practice is called the _____.

5. An order from a licensed veterinarian to a pharmacist is a _____.

6. Written information pertaining to past events of a patient is the patient's _____.

7. A detailed list of everything in stock in a practice is the _____.

8. What a patient pays an insurance company to insure a pet is the _____.

9. An official document signed by the veterinarian verifying vaccination is a _____.

10. The most commonly used medical record format is _____.

11. Loss of stock is referred to as _____.

12. Paying close attention to a client in communication is _____.

13. Showing understanding of a client's relationship to his or her pet is _____.

14. Summarizing what a client is expressing is _____.

15. Realization that the outcome of an event cannot be altered is _____.

16. The first stage of grief is _____.

N	I	R	T	R	U	M	M	P	G	L	S	G	A	E
M	O	E	E	L	E	U	K	N	D	H	Q	S	R	T
R	A	I	G	S	I	T	I	G	R	Z	V	S	T	A
M	O	P	T	M	O	T	U	I	A	K	W	T	N	C
K	T	R	E	P	A	L	N	P	L	C	I	I	E	I
O	S	R	E	D	I	K	U	R	M	O	P	N	I	F
U	P	F	I	C	A	R	H	T	N	O	I	V	T	I
Q	C	L	E	G	O	K	C	P	I	S	C	E	A	T
B	A	A	E	G	Q	R	B	S	D	O	W	N	P	R
V	C	L	I	E	N	T	D	M	E	W	N	T	X	E
R	E	F	L	E	C	T	I	O	N	R	A	O	F	C
G	N	I	D	N	E	T	T	A	I	L	P	R	Z	S
R	P	D	R	X	Z	Z	H	Q	A	E	J	Y	L	K
L	A	G	V	V	N	J	D	G	L	L	E	D	F	Y

IDENTIFY THE EMOTION FROM BODY LANGUAGE

For each of the photos, identify which of the following emotions you think is being relayed. Write your answer on the caption line.

1. _____ Shock

2. _____ Joy or pleasure

3. _____ Concern

4. _____ Anger or frustration

5. _____ Disbelief

6. _____ Grief

7. _____ Loneliness

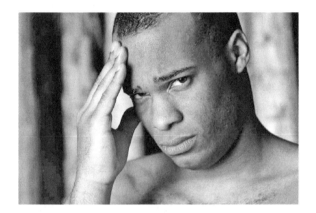

1. _____

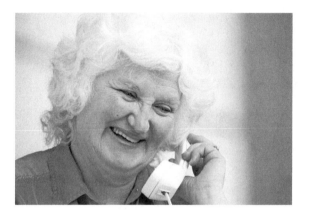

2. _____

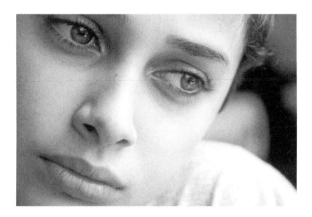

3. _____

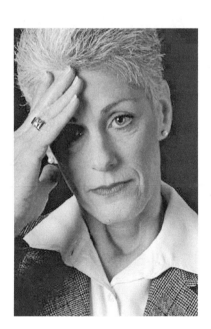

4. _____

15

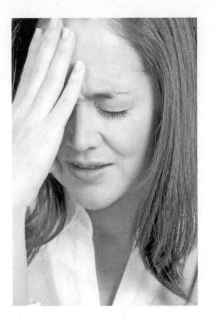

5. _____

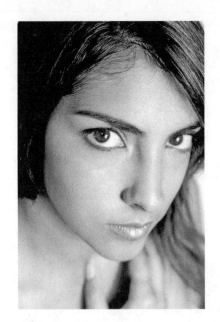

6. _____

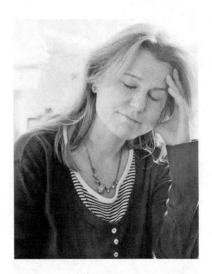

7. _____

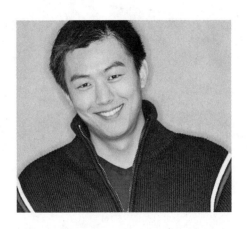

8. _____

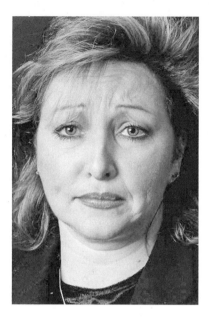

9. _____

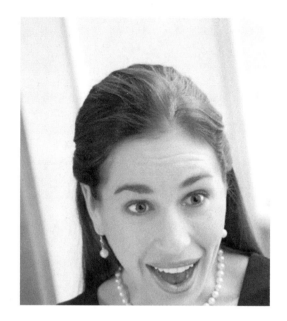

10. _____

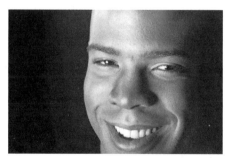

11. _____

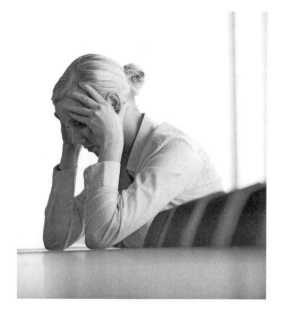

12. _____

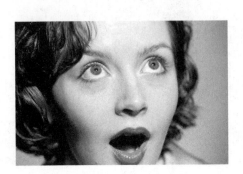

13. _____

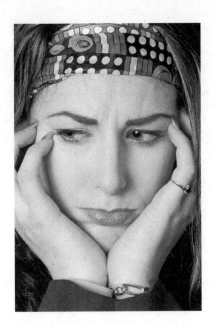

14. _____

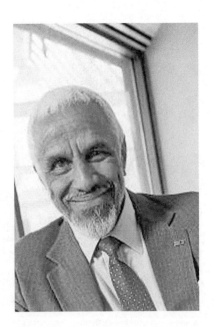

15. _____

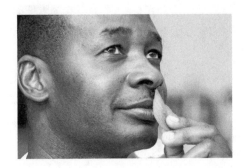

16. _____

CROSSWORD

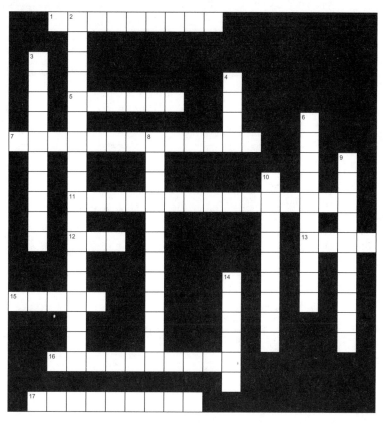

Across

1 Written _____ instructions provide the client with education on expected progression of illness or injury, treatment, care, use of medications, and follow-up

5 The cost of the product multiplied by a percentage

7 A legal document that must be complete, legible, and made available to clients at their request

11 Form signed by the client after all information regarding the procedure has been provided and the client has had the opportunity to ask questions

12 Standardized procedures in a practice, including check-in and release and record-keeping

13 Subjective observations, objective findings, assessment, and plan

15 The percentage of charges for which the owner is responsible after the deductible has been met

16 The amount an owner must pay before the insurance company will offer compensation

17 The loss of product without explanation

Down

2 Offers compensation for treatment of injured and sick pets

3 Summarizing what the client is expressing

4 A medical record that includes the defined database, the problem list, the plan, and the progress section

6 ___ fee covers the cost of the label, the pill vial, and the time used to count the medication

8 The level a stock item reaches before reordering

9 ___ release is a consent form that must state that the pet's death will result

10 The second-largest expense of the hospital

14 Certificate for ___ vaccination includes the client's name and contact information, patient's name, species, breed, gender, age, and vaccination information

Chapter **2** Office Procedures and Client Relations

3 Medical Terminology

LEARNING OBJECTIVES

After reviewing this chapter, the reader will be able to:

- Construct medical terms from word parts.
- Describe how to construct medical terms.
- Define the meanings of common prefixes and suffixes used in medical terms.
- Define terms used for common surgical procedures, diseases, instruments, procedures, and dentistry.
- Describe anatomic terms for direction.

DEFINITIONS

Give the meaning of the following word parts.

1. ex- _____

2. hyper- _____

3. pre- _____

4. dis- _____

5. dys _____

6. -gram _____

7. cardi- _____

8. peri- _____

9. -ectomy _____

10. tachy- _____

11. -rrhea _____

12. -pathy _____

13. -pexy _____

14. -plasia _____

15. -oma _____

16. -osis _____

17. -itis _____

18. -megaly _____

19. -tome _____

20. colp/o _____

MATCHING

Match the meaning with the prefix or suffix.

1. _____ -megaly   A. against
2. _____ hypo-   B. inflammation
3. _____ hydro-   C. hidden
4. _____ glycol-   D. state or condition
5. _____ -eu   E. enlargement
6. _____ anti-   F. slow
7. _____ -ize   G. normal
8. _____ -itis   H. sweet
9. _____ brady-   I. difficult
10. _____ -osis   J. use, subject to
11. _____ dys   K. water
12. _____ -crypt   L. insufficient

DEFINE

Indicate the correct combining forms.

1. Abdomen _____

2. Ankle _____

3. Chest _____

4. Bladder _____

5. Duct _____

6. Ear _____

7. Eye _____

8. Eyelid _____

9. Face _____

10. Fat _____

11. Foot _____

12. Gland _____

13. Hair _____

14. Lip _____

15. Mouth _____

16. Muscle _____

17. Nose _____

18. Spinal column _____

19. Spleen _____

20. Thymus gland _____

21. Toe _____

22. Tongue _____

23. Tooth _____

24. Uterus _____

25. Vein _____

MEDICAL TERMS

Give the correct medical term for each.

1. Before birth _____

2. Little urine _____

3. Excessive eating _____

4. Difficult breathing _____

5. Excessively slow heart rate _____

6. Out of place _____

7. Pertaining to throughout the entire animal kingdom _____

8. Not enough red blood cells _____

9. Difficulty swallowing _____

10. New tissue growth _____

11. Examination of a dead animal _____

12. Inability to move one side of the body _____

13. Long headed _____

14. Study of the endocrine system _____

15. Sugar in the urine _____

16. Inducing death painlessly _____

17. To make free from infection _____

18. Excessively fast heart rate _____

19. The plural of phalanx _____

20. Body temperature higher than normal _____

DEFINITIONS

Give the meaning of the underlined word part:

1. para<u>plegia</u> _____

2. <u>hemato</u>crit _____

3. anesthe<u>tize</u> _____

4. gastro<u>pexy</u> _____

5. herniorrhaphy   _____

6. colostomy   _____

7. abdominocentesis   _____

8. laparotomy   _____

9. cheiloplasty   _____

10. cholecystectomy   _____

Give the meaning of the following word parts:

1. Nephrosis   nephr/o: _____

    osis: _____

2. Leiomyoma   leiomy: _____

    oma: _____

3. Cardiology   cardi/o: _____

    logy: _____

4. Anaplasia   ana: _____

    plasia: _____

5. Carcinogenesis   carcin/o: _____

    genesis: _____

6. Tonsillitis   tonsil: _____

    itis: _____

7. Myalgia   my: _____

    algia: _____

8. Rhinoplasty   rhino: _____

    plasty: _____

9. Panzootic   pan: _____

    zootic: _____

10. Hematuria   hemat/o: _____

    uria: _____

11. Photophobia   photo: _____

    phobia: _____

12. Cardiomegaly   cardi/o: _____

    megaly: _____

13. Dyspnea   dys: _____

    pnea: _____

14. Diarrhea   dia: _____

                     rrhea: _____

15. Hydrocephalus   hydro: _____

                     cephalus: _____

MULTIPLE CHOICE

1. The term for toward the midline is:
   a. medial.
   b. lateral.
   c. proximal.
   d. distal.

2. The paw is _____ to the shoulder.
   a. cranial
   b. caudal
   c. distal
   d. proximal

3. Gastroplasty contains the suffix that means:
   a. excision.
   b. forming an opening.
   c. surgical repair.
   d. incision.

4. An incision into the duodenum is a:
   a. duodenectomy.
   b. duodenoscopy.
   c. duodenostomy.
   d. duodenotomy.

5. Which terms pertain to the tongue?
   a. lingual and gingival
   b. lingual and glossal
   c. lingual only
   d. gingival and glossal

6. Cystotomy is:
   a. resection of the urinary bladder.
   b. incision of the urinary bladder.
   c. inflammation of the urinary bladder.
   d. herniation of the urinary bladder.

7. Polyuria:
   a. is an abbreviated way of saying renal failure.
   b. is the opposite of anuria.
   c. means having more than one kidney.
   d. means having multiple pouches developing from the urinary bladder.

8. Nephromegaly is:
   a. inflammation of the kidney.
   b. suturing of the kidney.
   c. constriction of the kidney.
   d. enlargement of the kidney.

9. The term *angiorrhaphy* means:
   a. fixation of the vessels.
   b. suturing of the vessels.
   c. replacement of the vessels.
   d. destruction of the vessels.

10. A nasal discharge is referred to as:
    a. rhinitis.
    b. rhinorrhea.
    c. rhinorrhagia.
    d. epistaxis.

11. The surgical incision into the chest wall is known as:
    a. thoracentesis.
    b. thoracostomy.
    c. thoracotomy.
    d. thoracectomy.

12. The plural of fistula is:
    a. fistulare.
    b. fistulae.
    c. fistule.
    d. fistulus.

13. A benign growth of fat cells is a(n):
    a. lipoma.
    b. liposarcoma.
    c. adipocarcinoma.
    d. adiposarcoma.

14. Dead tissue is said to be:
    a. necrotic.
    b. plantigrade.
    c. polled.
    d. exfoliative.

15. The correct term for removal of the thyroid gland is:
    a. thyroidotomy.
    b. thyroidectomy.
    c. thyroplasty.
    d. thyroplegia.

16. Disease of the adrenal glands is termed:
    a. adrenal pathogen.
    b. adrenopathy.
    c. adenopathy.
    d. adenosis.

17. The plural of stimulus is:
    a. stimulum.
    b. stimulae.
    c. stimula.
    d. stimuli.

18. The term *ectopic* means:
    a. in the usual location.
    b. outside the usual place.
    c. outside the uterus.
    d. outside the reproductive system.

19. Inflammation of the outer ear is called:
    a. otitis externa.
    b. otitis media.
    c. otitis interna.
    d. panotitis.

20. The plural of cranium is:
    a. craniae.
    b. crania.
    c. cranius.
    d. craniora.

21. The prefix for "down, under, lower, against" is:
    a. cata-.
    b. andro-.
    c. ana-.
    d. cart-.

22. Which of the following suggests "lesser, decreased"?
    a. hyper-
    b. super-
    c. hypo-
    d. ultra-

23. Which of the following terms means an instrument for cutting the stomach?
    a. gastrotomy
    b. gastrotome
    c. gastroscopy
    d. gastroscope

24. Which of the following terms means partial paralysis of the stomach?
    a. gastrodynia
    b. gastroplegia
    c. gastromegaly
    d. gastrorrhexis

25. Which of the following terms means suturing a divided nerve?
    a. neuroplasty
    b. neuropexy
    c. neurorrhaphy
    d. neuromegaly

26. The term *nephrotomy* means:
    a. surgical removal of the kidneys.
    b. a mouthlike opening into the kidneys.
    c. cutting into the kidneys.
    d. visual examination of the kidneys.

27. *Dysuria* means:
    a. deficient urine production.
    b. painful or difficult urination.
    c. blood in the urine.
    d. pertaining to urination.

28. *Polyphagia* means:
    a. decreased hunger.
    b. excessive eating.
    c. no eating.
    d. much drinking.

29. A cat was diagnosed with a urinary tract infection. The laboratory analysis MOST likely noted is:
    a. anuria.
    b. oliguria.
    c. pyuria.
    d. nocturia.

30. *Osteoarthropathy* means:
    a. disease of the bone and joint.
    b. abnormal condition of the bone and cartilage.
    c. swelling of the bone and joint.
    d. destruction of the bone and cartilage.

31. Which of the following means surgical removal of the gall bladder?
    a. cholecystectomy
    b. cystocentesis
    c. cholecystoplasty
    d. cholecystemia

32. *Cystocentesis* means:
    a. movement of the thorax.
    b. sensation of the bladder.
    c. abnormal condition of the abdomen.
    d. surgical puncture of the bladder.

33. Which one of the following terms is in the plural form?
    a. testis
    b. testes
    c. granuloma
    d. appendix

34. An abnormally rapid respiratory rate is:
    a. apnea.
    b. bradypnea.
    c. dyspnea.
    d. tachypnea.

35. *Polyuria* means:
    a. decreased urine production.
    b. blood in the urine.
    c. pain in the urethra.
    d. much urine.

36. Which term describes the machine that records electrical impulses from the heart?
    a. electrocardiogram
    b. cardiometer
    c. cardioscope
    d. electrocardiograph

37. Which of the following terms means paralysis of the eye?
    a. oculoplegia
    b. ophthalmoparesis
    c. otopexy
    d. blepharoptosis

38. *Pyelonephritis* means:
    a. specialist in the study of kidney disorders.
    b. a condition of the kidneys.
    c. inflammation of the renal pelvis.
    d. pain in the kidneys.

39. *Peritoneal* means:
    a. pertaining to the peritoneum.
    b. a condition of the peritoneum.
    c. inflammation of the peritoneum.
    d. a disease of the peritoneum.

40. The procedure in which a laparascope is used to view the abdominal cavity is referred to as:
    a. abdominoscopy.
    b. abdominometry.
    c. laparascopy.
    d. laparatomy.

41. Which of the following terms means disease of the hair?
    a. trichopathy
    b. pilosis
    c. trichoplasty
    d. pilosclerosis

42. Which of the following terms means surgical repair of the kidneys?
    a. nephrectomy
    b. renopathy
    c. nephrolithotomy
    d. nephroplasty

43. *Myositis* means:
    a. inflammation of the muscles.
    b. inflammation of the spinal cord.
    c. a condition of the muscles.
    d. a condition of the spinal cord.

44. The arrectores pilorum muscles that attach to the hair follicles:
    a. relax as hairs are pulled more upright.
    b. cool the animal.
    c. are the singular form, whereas arrector pili is plural.
    d. are part of the sympathetic nervous system.

CROSSWORD

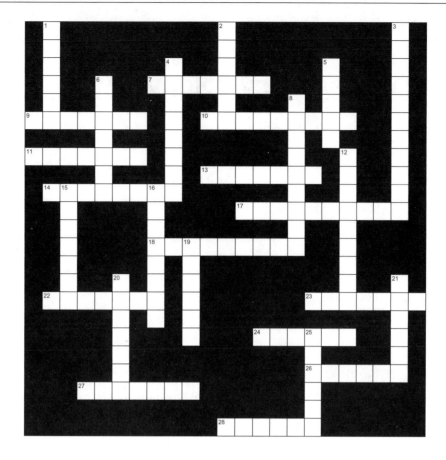

Across

7 Pertaining to the cranium or head end of the body
9 Pertains to the undersurface of the rear foot
10 Lying down
11 Pertaining to the nose end of the head or body
13 Tooth surface facing an adjacent or opposing tooth
14 The chewing or biting surface of teeth
17 Pertaining to or situated near the periphery
18 Movement of a limb or part toward the median
22 The act of bending, such as a joint
23 Pertaining to the underside of a quadruped
24 Pertains to the undersurface of the front foot
26 Pertaining to the back area of a body
27 At an angle, or pertaining to an angle
28 Tooth surface closest to the midline of the dental arcade

Down

1 Toward the cheek
2 Lying face up
3 Situated near the surface of the body
4 Nearer to the center of the body, relative to another body part
5 Lying face down
6 Denoting a position farther from the median plane of the body
8 Movement of a limb or part away from the median line
12 The act of straightening
15 Pertaining to or situated near the more proximal areas of the body
16 Next to, adjoining, or close
19 Farther from the center of the body, relative to another body part
20 Tooth surface toward the tongue
21 Pertaining to the tail end of the body
25 Denoting a position closer to the median plane of the body

Chapter **3** Medical Terminology

Anatomy and Physiology

LEARNING OBJECTIVES

After reviewing this chapter, the reader will be able to:

■ Describe types of cells and tissues of the body.
■ List the names of organs and structures that make up the various body systems.
■ Describe the ways in which organs and body systems function and interact.
■ Describe the general and special senses of the body and their functions.
■ Differentiate between exocrine and endocrine glands.

FILL IN THE BLANK

1. Cells are the _____ and _____ units of life.

2. Indicate with an arrow, the direction of the support relationship in the following formula:

   Cell Health _____ Tissue Health _____ Organ Health _____ System Health _____ Body Health.

3. Glandular epithelial cells secrete substances **directly** or **indirectly** (circle one) into the bloodstream.

4. The purpose of connective tissue is to _____.

5. Adipose connective tissue consists of _____.

6. Loose connective tissues include _____ fibers, reticular fibers, and elastic fibers.

7. Reticular fibers form a _____.

8. Elastic fibers provide some degree of _____.

9. Long bones have two extremities: _____ and _____.

10. Flat bones provide maximum area for _____.

11. The largest sesamoid bone is the _____.

12. Most of the bones of a bird are _____ bones because they _____.

13. The surface at which a bone forms a joint with another bone is the _____.

14. A condyle is usually found on the _____.

15. A hole in a bone through which blood vessels and nerves pass is a _____.

16. A fossa is a _____, usually occupied by a muscle or tendon.

17. A lump or bump on the surface of a bone is called a _____.

18. The bones found in the neck region are the _____.

19. The thoracic vertebrae are found _____.

20. The hind limb is termed the _____.

21. The thoracic limb is the _____.

22. The carpus is located between _____.

23. The purpose of the patella is to _____.

24. The _____ is the main weight-bearing bone of the distal leg.

25. The _____ in an animal is equivalent to the human ankle.

26. An example of a fibrous joint is _____.

27. Feathers and scales are part of the _____ in the nonmammalian species.

28. The largest organ in the body is the _____.

29. An albino animal has a total lack of _____.

30. Hair follicles, sebaceous glands, sudoriferous glands, and arrector pili muscles are found in the _____ of the skin.

31. The largest and main artery of the heart is the _____.

32. The mitral valve guards the atrioventricular opening in the _____ ventricle.

33. _____ immunity is the production of a specific antibody.

34. The primary function of the respiratory system is _____.

35. The _____ supplies the lungs with relatively pure, warm, humidified air.

36. The tooth root, which helps anchor the tooth in its bony socket, is covered by _____.

37. The two hormones produced by the pancreas are _____ and _____.

38. The cerebral cortex consists of _____ matter.

39. The medulla consists of _____ matter.

40. There are _____ pairs of cranial nerves.

41. The "fight-or-flight" reaction is produced by the _____ nervous system.

42. The "rest-and-restore" response is produced by the _____ nervous system.

43. Bitches come into season about once every _____ months.

44. The cat is an _____ ovulator.

45. The period of time from fertilization to delivery is called the _____ period.

LISTS

1. List the four basic tissues that make up the animal body:

   1. _____

   2. _____

   3. _____

   4. _____

2. All epithelial tissue share three common features. List them:

   1. _____

   2. _____

   3. _____

   _____

3. List the five glands that secrete directly into the bloodstream:

   1. _____

   2. _____

   3. _____

   4. _____

   5. _____

4. List the six types of connective tissue:

   1. _____

   2. _____

   3. _____

   4. _____

   5. _____

   6. _____

5. What are the three types of fibers found in loose connective tissue?

   1. _____

   2. _____

   3. _____

6. List the types of bones found in the mammal skeleton and give one example of each:

   1. _____   _____

   2. _____   _____

   3. _____   _____

   4. _____   _____

   5. _____   _____

7. List the bones of the pelvic limb from proximal to distal:

   1. _____

   2. _____

   3. _____

   4. _____

   5. _____

   6. _____

   7. _____

   8. _____

8. The axial skeleton comprises what four bones?

   1. _____

   2. _____

   3. _____

   4. _____

9. List the three pairs of bones that make up the pelvis in the adult animal:

   1. _____

   2. _____

   3. _____

10. List the three main types of joints and their movement:

   1. _____   _____

   2. _____   _____

   3. _____   _____

11. Synovial joints allow for six potential joint movements. List them:

   1. _____

   2. _____

   3. _____

   4. _____

   5. _____

   6. _____

12. What are five functions of the integument?

   1. _____

   2. _____

   3. _____

   4. _____

   5. _____

13. List the two main divisions of the circulatory system, their purpose, and the vessels contained in each:

	Purpose	**Vessels**
1. _____	_____	_____
2. _____	_____	_____

14. Breathing is controlled by two systems. List them:

   1. _____

   2. _____

15. List the three segments of the small intestine:

    1. _____

    2. _____

    3. _____

16. List the three important functions of the liver:

    1. _____

    2. _____

    3. _____

17. List the three divisions of the nervous system:

    1. _____

    2. _____

    3. _____

18. List the three types of muscles:

    1. _____

    2. _____

    3. _____

19. List the five senses:

    1. _____

    2. _____

    3. _____

    4. _____

    5. _____

20. List and define the special senses and where the cells are located:

    1. _____ _____ _____

    2. _____ _____ _____

    3. _____ _____ _____

    4. _____ _____ _____

    5. _____ _____ _____

21. List the major glands of the endocrine system and their function:

    1. _____ _____

    2. _____ _____

    3. _____ _____

    4. _____ _____

    5. _____ _____

    6. _____ _____

    7. _____ _____

Chapter **4** **Anatomy and Physiology**

22. List the components of the male reproductive system:

1. _____

2. _____

3. _____

4. _____

5. _____

23. List the components of the female reproductive system:

1. _____

2. _____

3. _____

4. _____

5. _____

6. _____

24. List the stages of estrus and a brief description of each:

1. _____   _____

2. _____   _____

3. _____   _____

4. _____   _____

5. _____   _____

TRUE OR FALSE

1. _____ The number of incisor and canine teeth in a dog and cat are identical.

2. _____ The most common dental problem in dogs and cats older than 5 years is periodontitis.

3. _____ Ova are continuously produced and are sloughed if not fertilized.

4. _____ Bone is second only to tooth enamel in hardness.

5. _____ Dogs have four digits in the forelimb; cats have five.

6. _____ Cartilaginous joints do not allow for any movement.

7. _____ A hoof is made of the surface layer of the epidermis.

8. _____ Sebaceous glands are sweat glands.

9. _____ Cats have only a few clustered sebaceous glands.

10. _____ A subcutaneous injection is administered in the hypodermis or subcutis layer of the loose connective tissue.

11. _____ The visible part of the hair is termed the hair follicle.

12. _____ The main purpose of erecting the hair is to make an animal warmer.

13. _____ The heart is a one-way pumping station that moves blood around the body.

14. _____ The tricuspid valve is located in the right ventricle.

15. _____ The placenta is connected to the fetus by the uterus.

16. _____ The larynx sits at the junction of the palatine tonsil and the epiglottis.

17. _____ A gunshot wound in the thoracic cavity can cause a collapsed lung.

18. _____ Each renal corpuscle is composed of glomeruli surrounded by a nephron.

19. _____ The large intestine absorbs water from the chyme.

20. _____ Most of digestion occurs in the stomach.

21. _____ The medulla is the largest part of the brain.

22. _____ The lens controls the size of the iris of the eye.

23. _____ The urinary system is the main system by which waste products are removed from the blood.

24. _____ Urine is transported to the urinary bladder by the ureters.

25. _____ Most parts of the reproductive system are not essential to life.

26. _____ To produce viable spermatozoa, the testes must be maintained at slightly higher than body temperature.

27. _____ Sperm are continuously produced and die in the epididymis if not ejaculated.

28. _____ Small-breed dogs reach puberty earlier than large dogs.

29. _____ Mammary glands are found in both males and females.

CROSSWORD

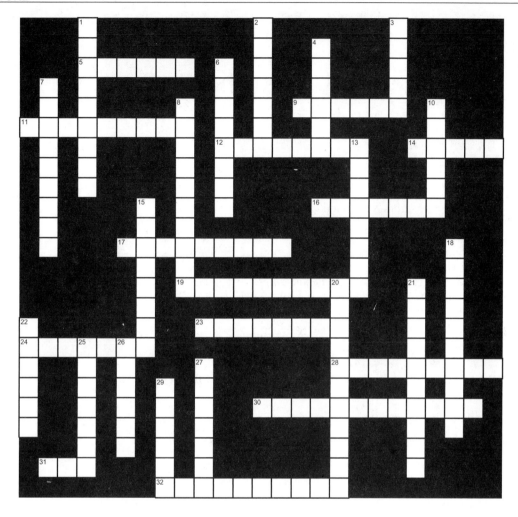

Across

5 A lymphoid organ, helps to "jump-start" the immune system; shrinks at sexual maturity

9 Transports urine from the renal pelvis to the urinary bladder

11 Meat eater

12 Life support system of a fetus

14 The longest cranial nerve

16 Carries urine from the urinary bladder to outside the body

17 Gland that produces tears

19 White blood cells

23 What a lymphocyte produces in the presence of a foreign body

24 Contraction of the heart chambers

28 Plant eater

30 Cell eating

31 A common congenital abnormality in dogs

32 Primary cellular component of the antibody-producing system

Down

1 Parturition in a cat

2 Responsible for the sense of hearing

3 Largest gland in the body

4 Cells that respond to stimuli and conduct impulses from one part of a cell to another

6 Parturition in a bitch

7 Dome-shaped muscle that separates the thoracic cavity from the abdominal cavity

8 A scavenger cell that will destroy foreign substances

10 Fluid portion of blood

13 The actual site of gas exchange in the lungs

15 Relaxation of the heart chambers

18 Responsible for the red color of blood

20 Red blood cell

21 A protein in plasma that forms a blood clot

22 Heat

25 Windpipe

26 Voice box

27 Houses the testes

29 Hardest substance in the body

Chapter **4** **Anatomy and Physiology**

5 | Pharmacology and Pharmacy

LEARNING OBJECTIVES

After reviewing this chapter, the reader will be able to:

- List the various categories of drugs and their clinical uses.
- Identify dosage forms in which drugs are available.
- Calculate drug dosages.
- List and compare routes by which various types of drugs are administered.
- Describe ways in which drugs exert their effect and affect body tissue.
- Explain procedures used to safely store and handle drugs.
- List the primary drugs affecting various body systems.

FILL IN THE BLANK

1. An example of a drug that can be inactivated by violent shaking of the vial is _____.

2. **TRUE OR FALSE (circle one)**: Dead space will cause the controlled substance log book to reflect more controlled substances than is actually in the vial.

3. Tuberculin and insulin syringes are available with attached _____ -gauge needles.

4. The larger the gauge number on a needle, the _____ the needle.

5. Needles larger than 1 inch are used for _____ and _____.

6. _____ medications may be supplied in single-dose vials, multidose vials, ampules, or large volume bottles or bags.

7. Drug control records must include receipts for purchase or sale of controlled substances and must be maintained for _____ years.

8. For veterinarians to legally use, prescribe, or buy a controlled substance from an approved manufacturer or distributor, they must have obtained a _____ number from the DEA.

9. The ideal range of drug concentration that minimizes detrimental effects and maximizes benefits is referred to as the _____ range.

10. A drug's _____ is the amount of drug administered at one time.

11. The time between administrations of separate drug doses is referred to as the _____ _____.

12. Parenteral drugs are administered by _____.

13. Per os drugs are administered by _____.

14. Topically administered drugs are administered by _____ them to the skin.

15. Injection of a drug outside the blood vessel is an extravascular or _____ injection.

16. Intramuscular (IM) administration involves injecting the drug into a _____.

17. Subcutaneous (SC or SQ) injections are administered under the _____.

18. Intradermal (ID) injections are administered within the _____.

19. Intraperitoneal (IP) injections are administered into the _____.

20. Drugs or functions related to the stomach are called _____.

21. Drugs or functions related to the small intestines are referred to as _____.

22. Drugs and functions related to the colon are termed _____.

23. Activated charcoal adsorbs _____ to its surface, preventing them from contacting the bowel wall.

24. Drugs that are used to induce vomiting are referred to as _____.

25. Overuse of _____ drugs can produce Cushing's syndrome.

26. _____ _____ is an injectable estrogen used after mismating in dogs.

27. To increase uterine contractions in animals with dystocia related to a weakened or fatigued uterus, the veterinarian commonly uses _____.

28. Drugs that kill or inhibit the growth of microorganisms or "microbes," such as bacteria, protozoa, viruses, or fungi, are called _____.

29. The ability to survive in the presence of antimicrobial drugs is referred to as *drug* _____.

30. The proprietary name of a drug is also referred to as its _____ name.

31. _____ are classified by generations, according to when they were first developed.

32. *Giardia* (giardiasis) is a protozoon that causes intestinal disease, and so _____ is a commonly used treatment.

33. Compounds that kill various types of internal parasites are called _____.

34. _____ interferes with development of the flea's chitin, which is essential for proper egg formation and development of the larval exoskeleton.

35. Drugs that relieve pain or discomfort by blocking or reducing the inflammatory process are called _____.

36. Both dogs and cats are very sensitive to the OTC NSAID medications _____ and _____, possibly developing liver and kidney failure; therefore, these drugs are not generally recommended for clients to give to their pets.

37. Metabolites of _____ can have severe side effects; a single extra-strength tablet (500 mg) can kill an average-sized cat and cause hepatic necrosis in dogs.

38. _____ is the destruction of pathogenic microorganisms or their toxins.

39. Chemical agents that kill or prevent the growth of microorganisms on living tissues are called _____.

40. Chemical agents that kill or prevent growth of microorganisms on inanimate objects are called _____.

41. The most common antiseptic applied to skin is _____ and usually is used in a solution of _____%.

42. A common quaternary ammonium compound used to disinfect inanimate objects in the veterinary clinic is _____ _____.

43. Two groups of chemicals broadly effective as disinfectants used on skin are _____ and _____.

44. The prefix that refers to 10^3 is _____ and is abbreviated _____.

45. The abbreviation for the prefix micro- is _____ and refers to a unit that is a power of 10 of _____.

1. Describe the differences between a nonproprietary (generic) drug name and a proprietary (trademark) drug name.

   _____

   _____

2. Drug manufacturers and distributors are required to identify a controlled substance on its label with a capital C followed by a Roman numeral, which denotes the drug's theoretical potential for abuse. Define the potential for abuse and provide two examples of drugs for each drug classification:

   C-I _____

   _____

   _____

   C-II _____

   _____

   C-III _____

   _____

   C-IV _____

   _____

   C-V _____

   _____

3. Pharmacokinetics involves absorption, distribution, metabolism, and elimination. Briefly explain what each of these entails and what organs, tissues, or vessels a drug interacts with on its journey through the body.

   Absorption

   _____

   _____

   Distribution

   _____

   _____

   Metabolism

   _____

   _____

   Elimination

   _____

   _____

4. Emetics are drugs that induce vomiting. Answer the following questions about emetics.

A. Specifically why are they used?

_____

_____

B. What hazard is associated with their use?

_____

_____

C. Under what circumstances should they not be used?

_____

_____

D. Which drug works well as an emetic in cats?

_____

_____

E. Which drug works well as an emetic in dogs?

_____

_____

5. What disadvantages are associated with using narcotics as an antidiarrheal?

_____

_____

_____

_____

6. Answer the following questions about laxatives, lubricants, and stool softeners.

A. What are the differences between irritant laxatives and bulk laxatives?

_____

_____

B. How does mineral oil work on the colon?

_____

_____

C. What does a stool softener do?

_____

_____

D. How does lactulose work?

_____

_____

7. List the components that the FDA states must be present on a drug container label.

_____

_____

_____

_____

8. Describe the difference between a productive cough and a nonproductive cough.

_____

_____

_____

_____

9. Why is it important to tell clients not to use OTC cold medicines for a cat's cough?

_____

_____

_____

_____

10. What are the insulins of choice for maintaining diabetic dogs and cats?

_____

_____

11. Estradiol cypionate is used on dogs to:

_____

_____

DOSAGE CALCULATIONS

1. A 6-lb cat is prescribed amoxicillin at 5 mg/kg twice a day for 7 days. The oral medication has a concentration of 50 mg/mL. How many milliliters will the cat need per day?

2. A 30-lb cocker spaniel is to get a ketamine and diazepam induction IV, and the dose is 0.025 mL/lb for each. How much ketamine and diazepam will you draw up?

3. A 44-lb dog requires amoxicillin. The veterinarian prescribes 10 mg/kg and the concentration is 100 mg/mL. How much amoxicillin will you give?

MATCHING—DRUG FORMULATIONS

Please match the description with the type of drug formulation.

1. _____ Solid dosage forms injected or inserted under the skin
2. _____ Tablets and capsules
3. _____ Drugs dissolve and release and are absorbed by intestinal wall
4. _____ Drug particles not dissolved in a liquid vehicle
5. _____ Solutions of drugs with water and sugar
6. _____ Administered via a needle and syringe
7. _____ Alcohol solutions meant for topical application
8. _____ Semisolid dosage forms that are applied to the skin
9. _____ Drugs dissolved in sweetened alcohol
10. _____ Drug dissolved in a liquid vehicle
11. _____ Semisolid dosage forms given orally

A. Ointments
B. Elixirs
C. Suspension
D. Implants
E. Tinctures
F. Solution
G. Injectables
H. Solid dosage forms
I. Pastes
J. Syrups
K. Suppositories

MATCHING—ANTIEMETICS

Match the drug name with the brand name.

1. _____ Phenothiazine tranquilizers
2. _____ Meclizine
3. _____ Prochlorperazine
4. _____ Metoclopramide
5. _____ Chlorpromazine
6. _____ Diphenhydramine
7. _____ Dimenhydrinate
8. _____ Cisapride

A. Compazine
B. Dramamine
C. PromAce
D. Propulsid
E. Reglan
F. Benadryl
G. Thorazine
H. Bonine

MATCHING—ANESTHETICS

Match the drugs with their effects and uses.

1. _____ Cough control; treatment of GI-related and colic pain
2. _____ Long-term control of seizures; euthanasia
3. _____ Reversal of CNS depression from xylazine and dexmedetomidine
4. _____ Inhalant anesthetic
5. _____ Commonly used dissociative anesthetic
6. _____ A strong narcotic analgesic, often on a patch
7. _____ CNS stimulant that increases respiration
8. _____ Calming effect; decreased stimulus response; light analgesic
9. _____ Benzodiazepine tranquilizer with good muscle relaxation
10. _____ "Laughing gas"—weak analgesic
11. _____ Phenothiazine tranquilizer—reduces anxiety
12. _____ Potent, with long duration of analgesia

A. Ketamine
B. Barbiturates
C. Nitrous oxide
D. Isoflurane
E. Acepromazine
F. Fentanyl
G. Diazepam
H. Xylazine
I. Butorphanol
J. Buprenorphine
K. Doxapram
L. Yohimbine

WORD SEARCH

Give the term for the following definitions and then find the terms in the Word Search below.

1. A drug dissolved in a liquid vehicle that does not settle out if left standing _____

2. A drug given intravenously as a single volume at one time _____

3. A drug in which the particles are suspended but not dissolved in the liquid vehicle _____

4. A drug that kills or inhibits the growth of microorganisms such as bacteria, protozoa, and fungi _____

5. A drug that paralyzes a worm but does not kill it _____

6. A drug that relieves pain or discomfort by blocking or reducing the inflammatory process _____

7. A reproductive hormone similar to progesterone _____

8. A solution of drug with water and sugar _____

9. A specific protein molecule on or in the cell that a drug will combine with _____

10. An alcohol solution meant for topical application _____

11. An altered drug molecule _____

12. An anthelmintic that kills worms _____

13. An order from a licensed veterinarian directing a pharmacist to prepare a drug for use in a client's animal

    _____

14. Another term for either antiseptics or disinfectants _____

15. Antimicrobial _____

16. Chemical agents that kill or prevent growth of microorganisms on inanimate objects _____

17. Chemical agents that kill or prevent the growth of microorganisms on living tissue _____

18. Compounds that increase the fluidity of mucus in the respiratory tract by generating liquid secretions by respiratory tract cells _____

19. Directly neutralize acid molecules in the stomach or rumen _____

20. Drugs that increase urine formation and promote water loss _____

21. Drug that inhibits bronchoconstriction _____

22. Drug that reduces swelling of mucous membranes _____

23. Drugs or functions related to the colon _____

24. Drugs or functions related to the duodenum, jejunum, or ileum (small intestine) _____

25. Drugs or functions related to the stomach _____

26. Drugs that are used to control seizures _____

27. Drugs that induce vomiting _____

28. Drugs that reduce the perception of pain without loss of other sensations _____

29. General term used to describe compounds that kill various types of internal parasites _____

30. Given by injection _____

31. Glucocorticoid _____

32. How a drug moves into, through, and out of the body _____

Chapter **5** **Pharmacology and Pharmacy**

33. Inhibits bacterial replication _____

34. Inhibits protozoal replication _____

35. Kills bacteria _____

36. Kills fungi _____

37. Kills viruses _____

38. Movement of drug molecules from the site of administration into the systemic circulation _____

39. Opens (dilates) constricted vessels _____

40. Protein hormones secreted by gonadotrope cells of the pituitary gland including FSH and LH _____

41. Size, frequency, and number of doses _____

42. Solution of drug dissolved in sweetened alcohol _____

43. Steroid hormones produced by the adrenal cortex of animals _____

44. The alteration of a drug by the body before being eliminated _____

45. Without a trademark or brand name; nonproprietary _____

```
C P M B Q L N B S T S C I T P E S I T N A T S Y E
I B R O B A S A A A N T I B I O T I C G B U D R M
R O W E P D N C X C T A R C G H E K M N S K I O I
E L N F S I M T N A T O T E I M Z S B P F M S T T
N U V S T C V E E G N E V S E R C I E E R T I A L
E S W I B U R R T C R V R T E I T N P U S S N M A
G L Z T L R N I H A S O I I S G S S M H C X F M W
G E I O S I B O P C B C T E C I N I A I W S E A A
R L O X D V D S I T S O G A O I N O T G M T C L R
N P U Q I I U T M T I L L N L A D E C F J N T F D
O W S C L R E A S Y A O K I T I N A B E N A A N H
I U C A O R N T C N Y M N O T I D L L X D R N I T
T B T I U C M I A I R V R D K E Y O U X C O T I I
P O O I G K O C A N T I C O N V U L S A N T S T W
R E D I C I M R E V C A C D F P M U B A M C C N P
O D O S A G E K T S V A T F S S R C Z L V E O A A
S D I C A T N A C I M E T S Y S N O N H U P L L R
B R E C E P T O R R C B R I I D S A G H R X O A E
A C I R E T N E A E E O M M N O O L R E T E N I N
U T A B X L I H V X H P I W I C Z O A T S H I C T
H Y B Z Z U P C K H G S T D I F T O I C O T C I E
A N T I M I C R O B I A L A S L U U T J G I I G R
D I O R E T S O C I T R O C B V Y G R O J I B N A
P G D I C I T N I M L W H T N A V D E E R X A U L
G O N A D O T R O P I N E N O S I T R O C P E F L
P U R Y S L A D I C I G N U F S O L U T I O N X Y
```

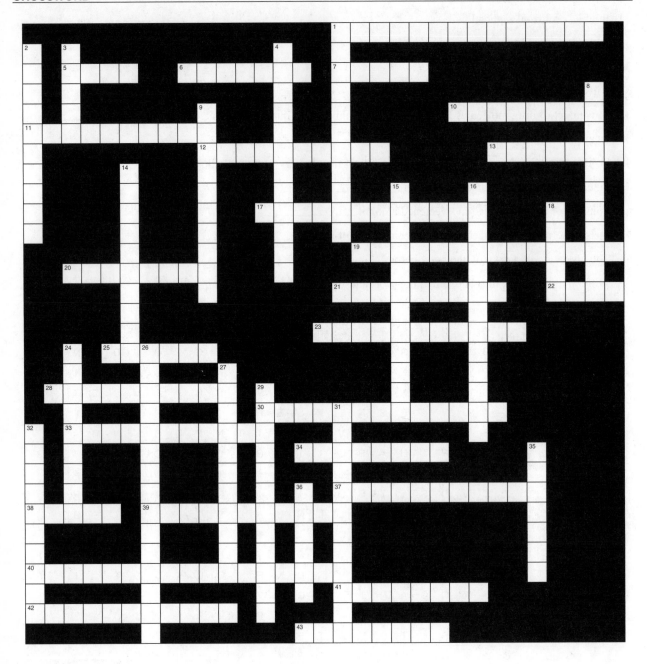

Across

1 A ___ level of a drug dose is below the ideal range of concentration, and therefore the beneficial effect is not achieved

5 Medications administered by mouth are ___ medications

6 A drug that is meant to be applied to the skin is a(n) ___ drug

7 A semisolid dosage form given by mouth

10 A drug dissolved in a liquid vehicle that does not settle out if left standing

11 A drug in which there are particles suspended but not dissolved in a liquid vehicle

12 Movement of drug molecules from the site of administration into the systemic circulation

13 The ___ name of a drug is also called its *nonproprietary* name

17 The movement of a drug from the systemic circulation into tissues

19 Anything that inhibits bacterial replication

20 A drug that increases urine formation and promotes water loss

21 Positive ___ drugs increase the strength of contraction of the heart

22 The amount of a drug administered at one time

25 A solution of a drug dissolved in sweetened alcohol

28 Any abnormal pattern of electrical activity in the heart

30 An injection made into a muscle mass

33 An injection made into a vein

34 The dosage ___ is the time between administrations of separate drug doses

37 A drug that increases the fluidity of mucus in the respiratory tract

38 A semisolid dosage form applied to the skin

39 An injection made within, not beneath, the skin

40 The alteration of a drug by the body before it is eliminated

41 An alcohol solution meant for topical application

42 Drug ___ is the removal of a drug from the body

43 The specific protein molecule on or in a cell with which a drug will combine

Down

1 A drug that is inserted into the rectum

2 A chemical agent that kills or prevents the growth of microorganisms on living tissue

3 A drug given intravenously as a single volume at one time

4 Anything that kills bacteria

8 Drugs that kill or inhibit the growth of microorganisms such as bacteria, protozoa, or fungi

9 Drugs that reduce the perception of pain without loss of other sensations

15 An injection made beneath the skin but not into a muscle

16 A term synonymous with antibiotic

18 The acronym for a nonsteroidal anti-inflammatory drug

24 A drug that paralyzes a worm but does not kill it

26 An injection made into the abdominal cavity

27 A drug that opens constricted vessels

29 A chemical agent that kills or prevents the growth of microorganisms on inanimate objects

31 General term used to describe compounds that kill various types of internal parasites

32 A drug that is administered using a syringe and needle is a(n) ___ drug

35 Drugs that function in the small intestines are ___ drugs

36 A drug that induces vomiting

6 Animal Behavior and Restraint

LEARNING OBJECTIVES

After reviewing this chapter, the reader will be able to:

- Describe the processes by which behaviors develop.
- Differentiate between positive and negative reinforcement and punishment.
- List and describe types of aggressive behavior that may be seen in dogs and cats.
- Describe the role of veterinary professionals in preventing behavior problems.
- List the steps in house training a puppy.
- Describe proper litter box care.
- List the different options cats look for in scratching posts.
- Describe the role of veterinary professionals in managing behavior problems.
- List and give examples of various behavior modification techniques.
- Describe the procedure for referring clients to professionals for resolution of behavior problems.
- Describe the psychological principles underlying physical restraint techniques.
- Explain and implement the safety precautions taken before and during physical restraint.
- Restrain dogs and cats for routine procedures such as physical examinations, nursing care, and sample collection.
- Give examples of behavior responses of animals to physical restraint.
- Correctly identify and use restraint equipment.

FILL IN THE BLANK

1. For any behavior to occur, there must be a _____.

2. Some problem behaviors are caused by _____ or _____ amounts of neurotransmitters.

3. The study of animal behavior is _____.

4. _____ conditioning refers to the association of stimuli that occur at approximately the same time or in roughly the same area.

5. _____ conditioning refers to the association of a particular activity with a punishment or reward.

6. The most important time period for behavior development in dogs and cats is _____ to _____ weeks of age.

7. Genetics can play a role in behavior problems, but _____ can also cause inappropriate behavior.

8. _____ reinforcement refers to any pleasant occurrence that immediately follows a behavior.

9. _____ reinforcement refers to any unpleasant occurrence that immediately follows a behavior and is used to create a desired behavior.

10. _____ is used to remove or decrease a behavior.

11. Positive punishment involves adding an _____ occurrence to decrease a behavior.

12. _____ punishment involves removing a desirable occurrence to decrease a behavior.

13. A delay of longer than _____ seconds between the behavior and the subsequent reinforcement significantly decreases the effectiveness of the reinforcement.

14. _____ refers to the attribution of human characteristics and emotions to animals.

15. Eight-week-old puppies cannot hold their bowels for longer than _____ to _____ hours.

16. One of the most important motivations for cats that scratch objects with their front claws is _____ marking.

17. The most common complaint from dog owners is aggression toward _____, whereas the most common complaint from cat owners is aggression toward other _____.

18. The sensitive socialization period in cats is _____ to _____ weeks.

19. In assessing a case of behavior problems, medical conditions that may account for the behavioral signs should first be evaluated; this is especially important with _____ and _____.

20. Behavior modification is needed to accompany _____ to increase the chances of a successful resolution of the problem.

21. _____ who meet the established criteria may be board certified by the American College of Veterinary Behavior and are considered behavior specialists.

22. The development of different breeds of animals is _____.

23. The _____ maintains a database of dog breeds.

24. An aggressive dog should be fitted with a _____ before entering the veterinary hospital.

25. For routine physical examination, cats can be restrained in _____ or _____ recumbency.

26. To restrain a cat, the practitioner uses the _____ restraint necessary and performs the procedure as _____ as possible.

27. One of the best tools for restraining a cat for venipuncture or injections is a large _____.

28. Never leave a cat on a tabletop inside of a _____ bag.

29. Sometimes it is possible to complete a procedure on a cat by puffing air in the animal's face; this is a _____ technique.

30. A very angry or wild cat can be sedated inside of a cage by squirting _____ into the animal's mouth.

31. A _____ is used to move an aggressive or fearful dog to or from a run or cage.

32. The _____ maintains a database of cat breeds.

33. What occurs during _____ or _____ can affect an animal for the rest of its life.

34. The best time to introduce animals to one another is when they are _____.

35. _____ conditioning can reinforce a good behavior.

36. Withholding attention from a jumping dog is an example of _____.

37. Aggression can be caused by a behavioral problem; it can also be caused by a _____ problem.

38. A leading cause of death in dogs and cats is _____.

39. **True or False** (circle one): Behavior problems are easier to correct than to prevent.

40. Unrealistic expectations occur when clients _____ their pets.

41. Most "accidents" with puppies occur when they are _____.

42. A decrease in chewing behavior can be accomplished with the use of a _____.

43. **True or False** (circle one): Physical punishment should never be used to correct house-training accidents.

44. **True or False** (circle one): Kittens need to observe the queen to properly use a litter box.

45. Cats prefer _____ substrates for elimination.

46. In a household with two cats, it is recommended that _____ litter boxes be available.

47. Front-claw scratching is a way of _____.

48. One of the most overlooked features when selecting a scratching post is the _____.

49. **True or False** (circle one): It is best to replace a well-worn, unsightly scratching post.

50. If a dog is caught chewing an unacceptable item, the owner should _____.

51. **True or False** (circle one): Aggressive behavior is normal in dogs and cats.

52. An injured dog should be transported using a _____, _____, or _____.

53. The way to calm a very nervous dog is to _____ and _____.

54. The _____ should extend past the end of the nose and should be snug but not constrictive around the neck.

55. One precaution in restraining a pregnant animal is to _____.

CIRCLE THE BEST ANSWER

1. Kittens **do** or **do not** (circle one) need to observe the queen eliminating in the litter box in order to know how to use it properly.

2. Studies have found that cats with elimination problems are more likely to have **scented** or **unscented** (circle one) litter as compared with cats without such problems.

3. It is recommended that in multiple-cat households there should be one litter box for **each cat** or **every two cats** (circle one) plus one.

4. The average age of young **boys** or **girls** (circle one) bitten by dogs is 5 to 9 years old.

5. **Male** or **female** (circle one) dogs are reported to be involved with 70% to 76% of all reported dog bites.

SHORT ANSWER

1. Give an example of positive reinforcement.

_____

_____

_____

2. Give an example of negative punishment.

_____

_____

_____

3. Describe how a person anthropomorphizes a pet's actions.

_____

_____

_____

4. When are the best times to take a puppy or dog outside to eliminate?

_____

_____

_____

5. Explain why the owner must go outdoors with the puppy to be successful in reinforcing elimination outdoors versus just waiting by the door.

_____

_____

_____

6. Give the general guidelines owners should know for maintaining a good litter box environment.

1. _____

2. _____

3. _____

4. _____

7. What unexpected result may happen if an owner catches his or her cat on the litter box in order to administer medications?

_____

_____

_____

8. The scratching objects must match the cat's preferences for the following criteria. Give a recommendation or an example for each criterion.

Desirable location

_____

_____

Height

_____

_____

Orientation

_____

_____

Texture

_____

_____

9. List four of the seven agonistic behaviors identified for both dogs and cats.

1. _____

2. _____

3. _____

4. _____

10. Give three examples of a variety of situations puppies and kittens should be exposed to in order to prevent fearfulness.

1. _____

2. _____

3. _____

11. What is the "fight-or-flight" principle?

_____

_____

_____

12. Describe the body language of dogs if:

Nervous

_____

_____

_____

Normal

_____

_____

_____

Aggressive

_____

_____

_____

13. What hazard is associated with gauntlets and restraint?

_____

_____

_____

14. Explain why you don't want to "puppy talk" when trying to get a dog to behave.

_____

_____

_____

15. Describe how to remove an aggressive dog from a run.

_____

_____

_____

16. Describe lifting a large dog from the floor to an examination table.

_____

_____

_____

17. What is counterproductive when restraining a cat?

_____

_____

_____

18. What is the body language of a cat that is trying to scare you off?

_____

_____

_____

19. Describe how a puppy test can be used to predict aggressive behavior in the adult dog.

_____

_____

_____

20. You have noticed that several clients are asking behavior-related questions that the veterinarian staff does not have adequate time to answer. What solutions could you suggest?

_____

_____

_____

21. Describe the steps in referring an animal to a behavior specialist.

_____

_____

_____

22. Briefly discuss the most common behavior problem in birds and small animals and why it occurs.

_____

_____

_____

23. Describe the best way to approach an unknown dog.

_____

_____

_____

24. Associate these dog behaviors with likely personality traits.

Wagging tail

_____

Ears drawn back, white of eyes showing, cowering

_____

Head lowered between the shoulders, level stare, and tail straight out

_____

25. Describe the precautions to observe when using an Elizabethan collar.

_____

_____

_____

_____

PHOTO QUIZ

Match the breed name with the correct image.

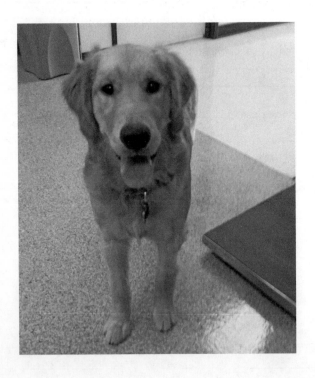

a. Papillon

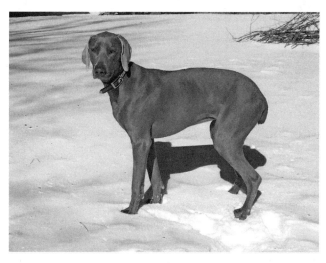

b. Beagle

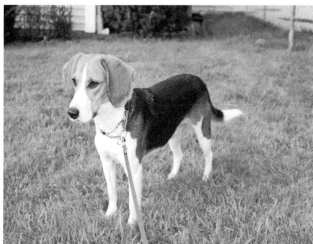

c. French bulldog

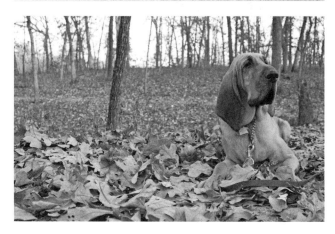

d. Australian shepherd

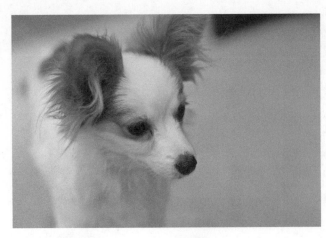

e. Bloodhound

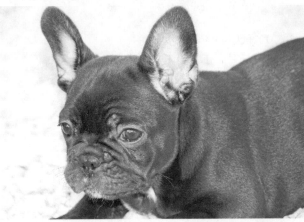

f. Weimaraner

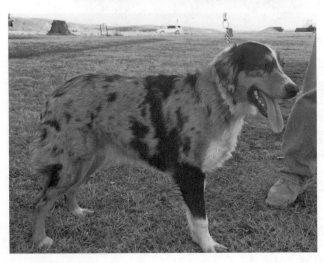

g. Shetland sheepdog

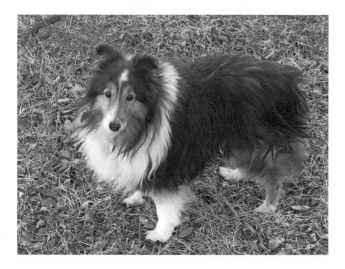

h. Golden retriever

MATCHING 1

Select the instrument that could be used to help restrain an animal for a procedure.

1. _____ Remove a shy or cowering dog from a cage

2. _____ Simple restraint

3. _____ Hissing, angry cat that is hiding under the refrigerator

4. _____ A growling dog with head down between the shoulders and with a level stare

5. _____ A dog with stitches

6. _____ An angry cocker spaniel (in the back room) that must be scruffed

7. _____ Removing an aggressive or fearful dog from a run

8. _____ A squirmy puppy

9. _____ Getting a blood sample from the femoral vein on a cat

10. _____ An injured dog

11. _____ Lifting an injured dog

A. Leash

B. Gauntlet

C. Capture pole

D. Muzzle

E. Restraint bag

F. Towel

G. Sedation

H. Elizabethan collar

I. Snuggle close to your body

Chapter **6** **Animal Behavior and Restraint**

MATCHING 2

Match the following procedures with the appropriate restraint.

Procedure

1. _____ Access to lateral saphenous vein
2. _____ Blood collection, cephalic vein
3. _____ Blood collection, jugular vein
4. _____ Cystocentesis
5. _____ ECG
6. _____ Enema
7. _____ Examine hind legs
8. _____ Examine a very large dog
9. _____ Examine a very wild cat
10. _____ Express glands
11. _____ IM injection
12. _____ IV injection
13. _____ Nail trimming
14. _____ Ophthalmic examination
15. _____ Oral examination
16. _____ Physical examination
17. _____ Radiographic procedure
18. _____ SQ injection
19. _____ Suture removal
20. _____ Taking a temperature
21. _____ Taking a pulse
22. _____ Taking respiration
23. _____ Urinary catheterization

Restraint

A. Cat lasso
B. Chemical restraint
C. Crowding
D. Dorsal recumbency
E. Inhalation chamber
F. Lateral recumbency
G. Standing restraint
H. Sternal recumbency

WORD SEARCH 1

Give the term for each definition, and then find the words in the word search below.

1. To take preliminary steps toward an animal _____

2. Danger _____

3. Any act done by an animal; exhibited for a reason and with purpose _____

4. Mechanical restraint device consisting of a metal pipe with a cable loop on one end _____

5. Mannerisms, postures, and facial expressions that can be interpreted as unconsciously communicating a person's or

    an animal's feelings or psychological state _____

6. An increase above the body's temperature caused by such things as drugs, toxins, or external temperatures, as in heat stroke _____

7. Feline restraint sack _____

8. Amount of restraint to use on a cat _____

9. Rigid pole with a loop at one end used to move an aggressive or fearful dog to or from a run or cage _____

10. Kind of behavior that is intended to harm another individual _____

11. Female animal parents, universally protective _____

12. Nylon, leather, or gauze covering placed over an animal's mouth to prevent biting _____

13. Exposure or liability to injury, pain, harm, or loss _____

14. A complex of all the attributes—behavioral, temperamental, emotional, and mental—that make each person and each animal unique _____

15. Protection from harm _____

16. Clinical term used to describe an animal lying down _____

17. A technique that uses mild pain to draw the attention of an animal away so a procedure can be performed _____

18. The state of being physically constrained _____

19. A dog's expression, exhibited by having ears drawn down and back, showing white around the pupils of the eyes, not making any eye contact, and cowering _____

20. Being held by the skin on the back of the neck _____

21. Attack _____

22. Restraint technique whereby an animal is held in position using a leash through a wall anchor or the hinges or the bars on a low cage _____

23. Escape _____

24. Heavy leather gloves used to restrain animals _____

25. Meekly obedient or passive _____

```
C  W  G  W  J  E  W  L  D  M  O  Y  K  J  U  N  C  W  S  F
F  H  M  N  L  R  U  M  R  R  M  G  F  Y  R  O  A  V  T  I
T  C  U  Z  I  F  F  Y  A  N  U  O  T  O  E  I  T  R  E  G
K  T  Z  T  R  B  X  N  Z  R  H  I  T  J  A  T  B  E  L  H
M  U  C  A  E  R  B  H  A  J  L  L  S  H  D  C  A  C  T  T
M  I  E  O  S  L  U  U  H  A  D  J  P  D  E  A  G  U  N  D
A  F  O  E  G  A  U  G  N  A  L  Y  D  O  B  R  R  M  U  F
A  I  Z  W  K  K  U  O  U  S  W  N  Z  W  Y  T  S  B  A  L
E  G  M  B  J  O  S  D  E  F  F  U  R  C  S  S  P  E  G  U
B  L  G  R  V  R  A  P  P  R  O  A  C  H  N  I  X  N  L  G
K  E  O  R  E  T  H  G  I  L  F  Z  J  I  U  D  I  C  Y  S
W  S  H  P  E  H  T  A  I  L  J  A  C  K  I  N  G  Y  T  T
G  M  R  A  H  S  T  O  C  K  S  I  N  Q  N  H  X  A  N  F
P  B  K  B  V  C  S  R  C  C  B  C  H  Y  O  S  N  I  E  L
V  B  X  F  M  I  T  I  E  C  C  B  R  G  W  C  A  D  S  A
E  D  E  Y  X  I  O  A  V  P  N  J  S  E  H  R  A  P  N  N
M  I  N  I  M  U  M  R  C  E  Y  N  X  I  T  N  E  M  E  K
E  V  I  S  S  I  M  B  U  S  A  H  O  S  G  L  H  S  F  I
M  S  H  W  T  U  S  B  Y  R  L  N  E  E  N  R  A  O  E  N
O  K  L  C  G  K  K  O  E  H  S  R  R  M  T  Z  X  H  D  G
```

WORD SEARCH 2

Fill in the blanks, and then find the words in the Word Search below.

1. To encourage a cat to play with an object, it can be scented with catnip or a commercial _____.

2. A veterinarian who is board certified in animal behavior by the American College of Veterinary Behaviorists

   _____

3. An internal or external change that exceeds a threshold, causing stimulation of the nervous or endocrine system

   _____

4. Any act done by an animal that is exhibited for a reason and with purpose _____.

5. Attributing human characteristics and emotions to animals _____.

6. Behavior that is intended to harm another individual _____.

7. Behavioral theory based on the principle that the consequences of a behavior will influence its frequency

   _____

8. Behaviors shown in situations of social conflict to diffuse aggressive behavior _____.

9. Exposure of a young animal to new experiences, people, other animals, and places with the goal of preventing

   fearful or anxious behavior in adulthood _____.

10. Female cat, intact; mother cat _____.

11. Material selected or preferred by an animal for urination and defecation _____

12. Passing of urine or feces _____

13. Rapid learning process that enables a newborn animal to recognize and bond with its caretaker _____

14. Something that decreases the likelihood of a behavior occurring _____

15. Something that increases the likelihood of a behavior occurring _____

16. The study of animal behavior _____

```
E  Z  S  G  M  N  A  N  H  E  U  M  Q  Y  O  B  E  H  A  V  I  O  R  P  T
N  L  D  O  E  J  N  B  U  E  L  S  E  Y  V  J  A  N  Z  H  D  O  W  N  U
O  S  O  C  I  A  L  I  Z  A  T  I  O  N  M  H  S  S  U  P  J  Y  E  O  X
M  R  R  S  S  W  T  Z  U  I  K  H  M  X  N  U  G  Z  N  I  M  M  C  H  C
O  F  A  M  Z  I  K  D  R  L  Y  P  I  I  W  W  T  V  W  K  E  W  M  G  V
R  J  D  Y  U  I  P  N  H  I  J  R  G  R  N  W  C  E  X  C  J  D  M  S  Z
E  G  I  X  S  K  Y  Q  M  G  G  O  L  H  B  A  U  J  R  K  J  W  J  A  D
H  E  N  T  F  P  Q  P  A  P  Z  M  D  V  J  M  T  O  N  A  X  S  S  E  R
P  Z  F  I  B  J  R  G  T  Q  A  O  A  J  H  V  F  I  R  M  E  Z  U  Y  L
C  X  S  D  N  I  F  J  B  Z  H  P  J  K  E  N  D  R  O  T  E  D  X  W  L
C  B  Q  Z  N  O  F  L  G  R  R  O  X  Q  I  S  F  O  A  N  E  S  R  B  F
L  F  K  T  N  I  I  F  R  H  U  R  Y  E  I  Z  C  R  F  H  W  H  H  C  L
Q  E  I  D  G  K  C  T  Y  V  T  H  R  Q  L  G  T  D  M  R  D  R  N  A  F
N  N  T  D  X  O  O  I  I  V  T  T  O  F  J  S  S  Z  O  O  N  A  E  H  U
G  U  R  H  E  W  K  L  T  D  F  N  H  X  B  U  T  R  J  M  Z  G  O  N  X
N  X  Y  O  O  Z  M  O  W  S  N  A  B  U  W  B  I  R  S  M  J  G  J  Y  F
H  R  G  Z  H  L  C  V  T  T  I  O  S  P  U  T  M  J  G  S  W  R  S  J  H
L  C  Y  N  E  X  O  B  X  F  T  N  C  W  U  V  U  F  O  K  Z  E  W  T  U
F  D  A  Y  C  X  U  G  L  J  D  J  O  T  F  V  L  R  H  M  I  S  J  U  E
V  R  X  F  X  Z  G  M  Y  O  V  M  T  G  N  B  U  U  X  Z  B  S  X  G  U
G  O  U  G  A  Z  O  Y  G  T  C  C  S  Y  A  A  S  E  G  J  W  I  W  X  Q
F  Z  Y  R  C  Y  K  L  Z  E  G  U  N  F  R  Z  R  L  W  K  X  O  X  U  H
T  S  I  R  O  I  V  A  H  E  B  Y  R  A  N  I  R  E  T  E  V  N  E  B  E
I  I  H  Y  D  C  P  H  H  T  N  E  M  H  S  I  N  U  P  B  V  E  R  H  Z
Q  V  J  K  K  L  Z  J  H  X  N  C  M  K  C  I  W  A  B  O  N  Q  Y  H  C
```

CROSSWORD

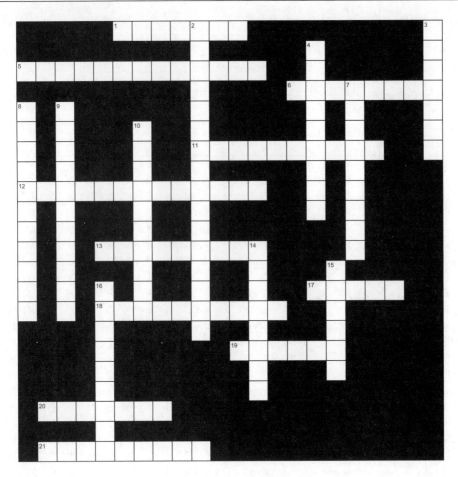

Across

1 ___ conditioning is a behavioral theory based on the principle that the consequences of a behavior will influence its frequency

5 Exposure of a young animal to new experiences, people, other animals, and places with the goal of preventing fearful or anxious behavior as adults

6 Any act done by an animal that is exhibited for a reason and with purpose

11 Something that decreases the likelihood of a behavior occurring

12 Something that increases the likelihood of a behavior occurring

13 Rigid pole with a loop at one end used to move an aggressive or fearful dog to or from a run or cage

17 An intact female cat

18 Behavior that is intended to harm another individual

19 ___ recumbency—restraint position whereby the animal is held in position resting on its back.

20 ___ recumbency—restraint technique whereby the animal is held in position resting on the side of the body

21 Material selected or preferred by an animal for urination or defecation

Down

2 Attributing human characteristics and emotions to animals

3 ___ recumbency—restraint technique whereby the animal is held in position resting on its breastbone

4 A natural or synthetic chemical that may influence an animal's behavior

7 Behaviors shown in situations of social conflict to diffuse aggressive behavior

8 A restraint technique that uses mild pain to redirect the attention of an animal so a procedure can be performed

9 Passing urine or feces

10 Rapid learning process that enables a newborn animal to recognize and bond with its caretaker

14 The study of animal behavior

15 A nylon, leather, or gauze covering placed over an animal's mouth to prevent biting

16 Heavy leather gloves used to restrain animals

7 Animal Husbandry and Nutrition

LEARNING OBJECTIVES

After reviewing this chapter, the reader will be able to:

- Discuss general housekeeping concerns in the veterinary practice.
- List basic energy-producing and non–energy-producing nutrients.
- Describe considerations for feeding young and adult dogs.
- Describe considerations for feeding young and adult cats.
- Discuss the fundamentals of exotic pet diet considerations.
- Explain nutritional peculiarities of livestock.
- Give examples of methods used in feeding livestock.
- Discuss basic differences in the digestive tracts of ruminants and monogastric animals.
- List and describe common diseases and ways in which they can affect people.
- Discuss methods used to control spread of zoonotic diseases.
- Explain the general principles underlying disease prevention.
- Discuss features of appropriate housing and nutrition for animals.
- List and discuss types of vaccinations and schedules of vaccinations for domestic animal species.
- Explain the principles of sanitation that relate to disease prevention.
- Describe factors that predispose to disease.

TRUE OR FALSE

1. _____ One of the most reliable methods of animal identification is the collar tag.

2. _____ Sanitization is the destruction of microorganisms and their toxins.

3. _____ A zoonotic infection is one that is hospital acquired.

4. _____ It is acceptable for clients to constantly change their cats' diets with various brands and types of commercial diets.

5. _____ Weaning of kittens should begin at 5 weeks of age.

6. _____ Feline urinary tract disease tends to occur more often in obese or sedentary cats.

7. _____ Domestic dogs do not need variety in their diets.

8. _____ Large-breed puppies should begin weaning at 3 to 4 weeks.

9. _____ Chemical agents that destroy pathogenic organisms are disinfectants.

10. _____ It is acceptable to mix chemical cleaners to increase their ability to provide a deeper cleaning, necessary in the veterinary environment.

11. _____ Petting and simple verbal praise are part of nursing care.

12. _____ Cow's milk is an acceptable substitute for mother's milk.

13. _____ Aging diminishes the sense of taste and smell.

14. _____ Children and the elderly are more susceptible to zoonotic diseases because their immune systems function at a lower level.

15. _____ Natural immunity occurs when maternal antibodies cross the placenta.

16. _____ Active immunity occurs when an animal develops antibodies on its own.

17. _____ It is recommended that the feline leukemia virus vaccine be given in the left forelimb.

18. _____ An average-sized dog is considered geriatric after age 15.

19. _____ One who studies diseases is a pathologist.

20. _____ Patients with a nasogastric tube require a soft diet.

FILL IN THE BLANK

1. An agent that causes an abnormal increase in body temperature is a _____

2. Water balance in the system affects the ability to excrete _____.

3. Anorexic patients are fed with a _____.

4. _____ must be based on age, breed, health status, activity level, and reproductive condition.

5. Allowing pets free access to food at any time increases _____, which leads to obesity.

6. Pet foods should be tested by the association called the _____.

7. Sick or injured pets need good nutritional support to counteract the immunosuppressive effects of _____,

   _____, _____, _____, and _____.

8. After feeding tube placement, the amount of food is gradually increased over 3 days with 5 mL of water every

   _____.

9. Evaluating tissues with a microscope is called _____.

10. Small stones composed of cellular debris and mineral crystals are _____.

11. The total daily fluid volume for maintenance TPN is _____.

12. Water-soluble vitamins are passively absorbed from the _____.

13. Orogastric intubation is excellent for rapid administration, but it can cause _____ and _____.

14. Gradual introduction of dextrose is needed to avoid _____.

15. _____ provides the foundation for metabolism of all the nutrients in the body.

16. _____ is added to the diet for the treatment of obesity.

17. Cats require _____ fatty acids in their diet.

18. Husbandry involves _____, _____, and _____ of animals.

19. The ambient room temperature in the veterinary environment should be kept at _____ to _____.

20. The general rule for a holding enclosure is a minimum of _____ times the body size of the animal.

21. _____ is the destruction of microorganisms or their toxins.

22. A ventilation system should be capable of exhausting all air within a building in _____ to

    _____ minutes to facilitate odor control.

23. A _____ is any constituent of food that is ingested to support life.

24. Two means of controlling intake of a pet's food are _____ and _____ control.

25. Weaning large-breed puppies begins at _____ weeks of age; smaller breeds, at _____ weeks of age.

26. The most common nutritional disorder of pets is _____.

27. Three routes of nutritional support are _____, _____, and _____.

28. Orphaned kittens should not be weaned until _____ weeks of age.

29. The end result of tissue repair is usually _____ or _____.

30. Highly vascularized connective tissue produced after extensive tissue damage is _____ tissue.

31. Organisms that can cause disease in a host are _____.

32. Bacteria are classified either as _____ or _____.

33. Diseases transmitted between animals and people are _____ diseases.

34. The infective agent in 50% of dog bites and 90% of cat bites is _____.

35. Cat bites are _____ more times likely to become infected than dog bites.

36. A sign of anal sacculitis is _____.

37. Inappropriate urination is one symptom of _____.

38. Swelling and a rapidly growing firm mass at the site of a recent vaccination in a cat is a common sign of _____.

39. Chronic infections of the oral cavity, skin, and respiratory tract; chronic fever; and cachexia in a cat are common signs of _____.

40. One sign of infectious canine tracheobronchitis (kennel cough) is _____.

MATCHING

Match the following items with the descriptions.

1. _____ Body conditioning score

2. _____ Forage

3. _____ By-product feeds

4. _____ Herbivore

5. _____ Obesity

6. _____ Portion-control feeding

7. _____ Free-choice feeding

8. _____ Time-control feeding

9. _____ Water

10. _____ Essential amino acids

11. _____ Nonessential amino acids

12. _____ Nutrient

13. _____ Carnivore

14. _____ Water-soluble vitamins

15. _____ Fat-soluble vitamins

A. Amino acid that is synthesized in the body

B. Meat eater

C. Vitamins absorbed from the small intestines—excess amount excreted in urine

D. Vitamins metabolized and stored in the liver

E. Plant eater

F. Method of subjectively qualifying body fat reserves

G. Residues of food-processing industry

H. Daily portion offered either in single feeding or divided into several portions

I. Foundation for metabolism of all nutrients in the body

J. Most common nutritional disorder of pets

K. Feeds made up of most or all plant

L. Access to food 24 hours a day

M. Amino acid that cannot be synthesized in the body

N. Any constituent of food that can be ingested to support life

O. Portion fed with access for only 10 to 15 minutes

65

LISTS AND SHORT EXPLANATIONS

1. List the six basic nutrients:

    1. _____

    2. _____

    3. _____

    4. _____

    5. _____

    6. _____

2. Name five dietary minerals named in this chapter:

    1. _____

    2. _____

    3. _____

    4. _____

    5. _____

3. What steps should be followed for time-controlled feeding?

    1. _____

    2. _____

4. List vitamins that may be required in older dogs:

    1. _____

    2. _____

    3. _____

    4. _____

    5. _____

5. Obesity may predispose pets to what three things?

    1. _____

    2. _____

    3. _____

6. Describe techniques used to enhance aroma and taste of food for cats:

    1. _____

    2. _____

    3. _____

7. Name three reasons that homemade diets are not always the best for a pet:

    1. _____

    2. _____

    3. _____

8. What does the acronym AAFCO stand for?

_____

9. Total parenteral nutrition is a practical alternative for patients with what four conditions?

   1. _____

   2. _____

   3. _____

   4. _____

10. Preventive medicine involves these three major components:

   1. _____

   2. _____

   3. _____

11. The type of food and feeding frequency are based on five factors:

   1. _____

   2. _____

   3. _____

   4. _____

   5. _____

12. A hospitalized patient is a candidate for nutritional support if the following occur:

   1. _____

   2. _____

   3. _____

13. List the fat-soluble vitamins:

   1. _____

   2. _____

   3. _____

   4. _____

   5. _____

14. Gross lesions are described by what five characteristics?

   1. _____

   2. _____

   3. _____

   4. _____

   5. _____

15. Diet selection used in enteral nutritional support is based on:

    1. _____

    2. _____

    3. _____

16. List four types of factors that predispose an animal to disease:

    1. _____

    2. _____

    3. _____

    4. _____

17. At a minimum, a hospitalized patient requires a record of what four findings?

    1. _____

    2. _____

    3. _____

    4. _____

MULTIPLE CHOICE

1. Which of the following is not an essential fatty acid in cats?
   a. linoleic
   b. linolenic
   c. taurine
   d. arachadonic

2. Energy is used for:
   a. metabolism.
   b. fighting disease.
   c. skin turgor.
   d. clotting.

3. Dietary protein is used for:
   a. digestion.
   b. metabolism.
   c. building body tissue.
   d. cell repair.

4. Cow's milk is not a proper substitute for mother's milk in neonatal puppies because it is lacking:
   a. glucose and phosphorus.
   b. protein and lactose.
   c. potassium and sodium.
   d. iron and selenium.

5. Diets for active dogs must have enhanced levels of:
   a. magnesium.
   b. selenium.
   c. fat.
   d. phosphorus.

6. Phosphorus should be limited in older dogs owing to detrimental effects on:
   a. liver.
   b. kidney.
   c. heart.
   d. lungs.

7. Prevention of uroliths involves manipulation of the dietary intake of minerals, water, and:
   a. fiber.
   b. vitamin A.
   c. vitamin C.
   d. fat.

8. Although canned food has greater palatability, its use raises some concerns for the health of the:
   a. kidneys.
   b. teeth.
   c. heart.
   d. lungs.

9. A patient is a candidate for nutritional support if the animal has:
   a. lost more than 10% of body weight.
   b. diarrhea with body-conditioning loss.
   c. organ dysfunction.
   d. all of the above.

10. The route of nutritional support can be:
    a. enteral.
    b. parenteral.
    c. intravenous.
    d. a and b.

WORD SEARCH

Fill in the blanks with the correct word and then find the words in the word search below.

1. Plant-eating animal _____

2. Organic compound made of chains of amino acids _____

3. Nutrient that contains more energy per unit of weight than any other _____

4. Route of delivery of nutrients directly into the stomach _____

5. Meat-eating animal _____

6. Building block of protein _____

7. Any constituent of food that is ingested to support life _____

8. An essential mineral _____

9. The process of converting food into chemical substances that can be absorbed into the blood and used by the body

   tissues _____

10. Organic substance found in foods that is essential in small quantities for growth, health, and survival

    _____

11. That portion of ingested foodstuffs that cannot be broken down by intestinal enzymes and therefore passes through

    the colon undigested _____

12. Given by injection _____

13. The set of chemical reactions that happen in living organisms to maintain life _____

14. Excessive accumulation of fat in the body _____

15. A dietary mineral that can have detrimental effects on the kidney _____

16. Organs that filter the blood and excrete the end products of body metabolism in the form of urine

_____

```
I  T  A  I  Q  L  A  R  H  L  A  T  O  P  P  U  N  V  W  H
L  L  L  L  A  C  H  R  A  I  M  N  Q  T  L  Q  X  K  E  D
P  U  N  D  F  D  G  R  Z  D  I  E  F  Q  P  R  D  R  M  N
N  H  U  O  F  A  E  Q  R  F  N  I  P  E  M  F  B  Q  N  R
B  W  O  P  I  T  L  R  I  X  O  R  M  N  E  I  J  L  X  J
S  Z  W  S  N  T  E  F  F  C  A  T  B  D  V  D  E  M  R  K
G  P  I  E  P  B  S  Q  A  C  C  U  V  O  T  J  I  G  L  M
O  A  R  X  I  H  D  E  Q  V  I  N  R  L  A  R  E  T  N  E
T  A  B  F  U  V  O  H  G  V  D  E  V  I  T  A  M  I  N  O
P  T  I  S  J  C  A  R  O  I  S  Z  V  K  C  R  D  Q  F  F
Z  N  Z  W  L  F  R  U  U  A  D  Y  Q  F  Y  F  G  A  V  A
W  R  A  G  X  B  R  E  Q  S  O  E  E  N  K  A  D  P  B  T
M  E  T  A  B  O  L  I  S  M  B  G  Y  N  D  T  R  Q  F  K
B  P  F  I  A  Z  K  Z  U  L  E  A  P  E  D  O  W  L  B  Q
E  M  Z  Q  C  N  U  I  W  U  S  R  H  F  T  I  S  Z  Y  U
Q  P  C  T  O  Q  N  W  Z  U  I  O  Q  E  E  N  K  U  U  O
Z  U  X  Z  O  E  X  H  X  U  T  F  I  I  W  V  J  X  S  V
C  V  T  L  L  K  T  R  V  U  Y  N  Y  F  G  T  W  M  N  R
X  V  C  E  F  O  R  C  E  R  O  V  I  N  R  A  C  L  N  Q
B  S  S  I  Q  B  P  E  S  S  I  H  V  D  V  I  G  Q  J  E
```

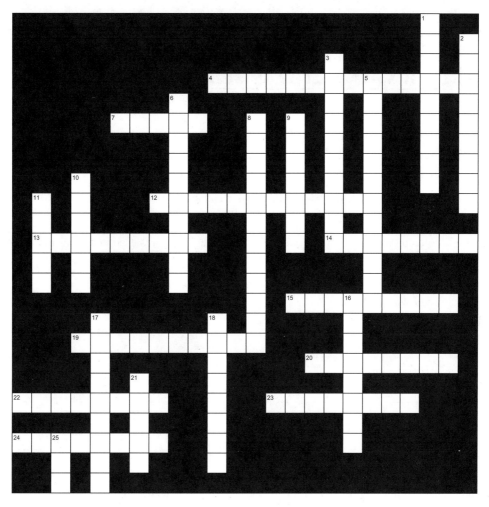

Across

4 A scoring method of subjectively quantifying subcutaneous body fat reserves

7 _____-soluble vitamins are passively absorbed from the small intestine, and excess amounts are excreted in the urine

13 A location in which a pathogenic agent is maintained before transmission

14 Any constituent of food that is ingested to support life

15 __ amino acids cannot be synthesized in the body and so must be supplied by the diet

19 A tear or jagged wound

20 Small stones composed of cellular debris and mineral crystals

22 Any disease or infection that is naturally transmissible between vertebrate animals and humans

23 Procedure performed on an animal after death to evaluate cause of death

24 An organism that causes disease

Down

1 The type of feeding in which food is offered at all times so the animal can eat at its leisure

2 Bruise

3 A violent shock or jarring of the tissue

5 The destruction of microorganisms and their toxins

6 Energy-producing nutrients have a hydrocarbon structure that produces energy through digestion, _____, or transformation

8 The reduction of the number of organisms to a safe level

9 The most common nutritional disorder in pets

10 Protein coat surrounding a virus

11 An extremely small, nonliving infectious agent that can cause disease in a wide variety of animals

16 The study of the cause of disease

17 The study of disease

18 Scarring; the end result of tissue repair

21 Fat-soluble vitamins are metabolized in a manner similar to fats and stored in the _____

25 Acronym for total parenteral nutrition

8 Animal Care and Nursing

LEARNING OBJECTIVES

After reviewing this chapter, the reader will be able to:

- Describe techniques used in the general nursing care of dogs and cats.
- Discuss techniques used in the recording of patient care.
- Describe procedures used in grooming and skin, nail, and ear care.
- List common routes of administration of medication, and describe procedures used in administration of medications.
- List and describe methods of parenteral administration.
- List and describe methods of intravenous catheterization.
- Explain the principles of first-aid treatment of wounds.
- Explain the principles of wound closure.
- Give examples of the types and application of bandages.

SHORT ANSWER/FILL IN THE BLANK

1. What are the foundations on which sound medical and nursing interventions are based?

   _____

2. What is the key to successful history taking?

   _____

3. The best clinical interview focuses on the _____.

4. Patients are evaluated using a combination of methods. These include which four methods?

   _____

   _____

5. List the vital signs recorded for every patient.

   _____

   _____

6. To take a temperature, leave the thermometer in the rectum for _____ to _____ minutes.

7. Shock, severe sepsis, severe cardiac insufficiency, multiple organ failure, and poor perfusion secondary to anesthesia

   or surgery or with low environmental temperatures can result in _____.

8. In patients with marked hypothermia, the rectal temperature should be monitored at least every _____ minutes.

9. Normal heart rates for cats and kittens range from _____ to _____ beats/min.

10. Normal heart rates for dogs range from _____ beats per minute in larger dogs to as high as _____ beats per minute in puppies.

11. Pulses can be described as _____, _____, _____, _____,

_____, or _____.

12. A transient murmur that often disappears by 3 to 4 months of age is termed _____ _____

_____.

13. The patient should be in _____ recumbency and allowed to inhale oxygen during the exam if stressed, to facilitate lung expansion and accurate auscultation.

14. Dyspnea may be manifested by _____ _____ _____ _____.

15. Normal urine output in dogs and cats is _____.

16. "Scooting" on the hindquarters and licking of the anal area are signs of _____ _____

_____ _____.

17. The anal sacs are emptied with the dog restrained in the _____ position.

18. _____ _____ of the anal gland is not recommended because of the frequent occluding of the ducts, inability to completely empty the sacs, and excessive pain it may cause the patient.

19. Signs of ear disease include:

_____

20. When giving a medicated bath or applying topical medication, the veterinary staff person should wear

_____ _____ and/or _____ _____.

21. An enema introduces fluids into the rectum and also stimulates _____ _____, as well as

evacuating the _____ _____ for diagnostic procedures, and irrigates the _____.

22. Enemas are contraindicated if the bowel is

_____

23. Intradermal (ID) injections are used primarily for _____ and _____ anesthesia.

24. Subcutaneous (SQ) injections are used for:

_____

25. When is the use of winged infusion (butterfly) catheters most appropriate?

_____

26. The reason the client has sought veterinary care for the animal is

_____

27. Patients are usually placed in _____ recumbency for urinary catheterization.

28. Securing the catheter reduces movement of the catheter in the vessel and can decrease the likelihood of

_____

29. Nasogastric tubes are inserted through the nares and through the _____ to the _____.

30. _____ _____ is one of the most commonly used supportive measures in veterinary medicine and is an important aspect of virtually every critical care case.

31. Wound assessment includes evaluation of the wound's

_____

_____

_____

_____

32. The term *euthanasia* is derived from the Greek *eu-,* meaning good, and *thanatos,* meaning

_____

33. Hyperthermia can be controlled with

_____

TRUE OR FALSE

1. _____ Elastic adhesive tape is compliant and applies continuous, dynamic pressure to the wound as the patient moves.

2. _____ Wet-to-wet dressings cause more pain and tissue damage than dry dressings when removed.

3. _____ Congenital and infectious diseases, parasitism, ingestion of foreign bodies, and intussusceptions are usually predominant in young animals.

4. _____ Debridement means the wound is free of bacteria.

5. _____ Regurgitation is the same thing as vomiting.

6. _____ The presenting complaint is what the client perceives the patient's problem to be.

7. _____ Medications given orally are metabolized instantly.

8. _____ Excessive nail length results in altered gait.

9. _____ With a standard mercury thermometer, the thermometer must be left in place in the rectum for at least five minutes.

10. _____ Silver nitrate may permanently stain countertops or exam tables.

11. _____ Patients with marked hypothermia should have their temperature checked and recorded at least every thirty minutes.

12. _____ Normal heart rates for cats and kittens range from 120 to 240 beats/min.

13. _____ Arrhythmias that are characterized by intermittent, prolonged periods of asystole are termed *bradyarrhythmias.*

14. _____ A normal sinus rhythm involves a difference in the pulse rate and heart rate when determined simultaneously.

15. _____ Innocent murmurs are usually only found in neonatal kittens and disappear before 4 weeks of age.

16. _____ Wound contamination is not the same as wound infection.

17. _____ Normal respiratory rates in small animals are approximately 18 to 30 breaths/min.

18. _____ Stridor is defined as a low-pitched snoring noise.

19. _____ For severe hyperthermia, apply isopropyl alcohol to the foot pads.

20. _____ Most ear cleaning solutions are ototoxic if the tympanic membrane is not intact.

SHORT ANSWER

1. Reflective listening skills are important in client interviewing. What is reflective listening, and why is it important?

_____

_____

_____

_____

2. What elements are important to record on an intake exam?

_____

_____

_____

_____

3. What does an evaluation of perfusion involve?

_____

_____

4. For a patient under care or treatment, what vital signs need to be recorded, and when?

_____

_____

5. What will trigger hyperthermia (abnormally high body temperature)?

_____

_____

6. What do brick red membranes indicate?

_____

7. What is the significance of cyanotic mucous membranes (blue colored)?

_____

_____

8. Why is it important to question geographic origin, prior ownership, and environment?

_____

_____

_____

9. Your patient says, "My dog just had a stroke." What should your first question be?

_____

_____

_____

10. Describe the basic technique for bathing dogs and cats.

_____

_____

_____

_____

_____

_____

_____

_____

_____

11. Some hospitalized patients develop skin problems (e.g., decubital ulcers, pyoderma, urine scald, dry scaly skin). Explain why this can happen.

_____

_____

12. Before the patient is discharged from the hospital, what routine procedures should be performed?

_____

_____

13. What technique should be used to avoid cutting pigmented (black) nails too short in a dog?

_____

_____

14. What would be included in a list of topical medications for use in a veterinary practice?

_____

_____

15. List common respiratory sounds.

_____

_____

16. Describe how to give a pill to a dog.

_____

_____

_____

_____

_____

_____

17. Describe how to give a pill to a cat.

_____

_____

_____

_____

_____

_____

18. List the parenteral routes of medication administration.

_____

_____

_____

19. For what purposes would an intravenous catheter be placed?

_____

_____

_____

20. Differentiate between a laceration and a contusion.

_____

_____

_____

_____

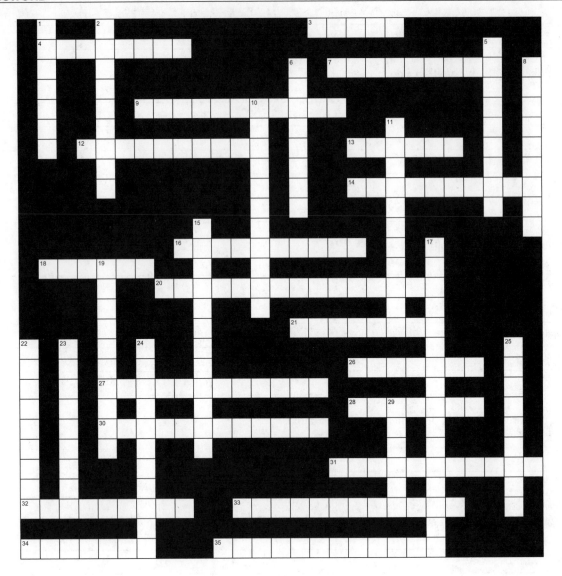

Across

3 Disruption of cellular and anatomic functional continuity
4 Straining to defecate
7 The mental state or status of a patient
9 Slower-than-normal heart rate
12 Separation of layers of a surgical wound
13 Tool used to ensure the nail bed is trimmed down without causing trauma or bleeding
14 Tapping of the body's surface to produce vibration and sound
16 Good death
18 To irrigate or wash
20 Pressure sores (bedsores) that result from an animal lying on a bony prominence for too long
21 Blue
26 Longstanding
27 Abnormally high body temperature
28 Low-pitched, snoring noise
30 Route of administration used to inject medication and fluids in pediatric patients
31 Faster-than-normal heart rate
32 Involuntary eye movement
33 Maintenance of normal body temperature
34 Increased respiratory effort or difficulty breathing
35 A surgical device placed in a wound to drain fluid

Down

1 High-pitched, harsh, wheezy noise
2 Lying down
5 Pain relief in the form of oral, transdermal, or injectable medication
6 Nail trimming
8 Respiratory distress exacerbated by recumbency
10 The lack of gas exchange within alveoli, usually caused by alveolar collapse or fluid consolidation
11 Excising dead and dying tissues
15 Listening to sounds produced by the body
17 Narrowing of the blood vessels
19 Irregular heartbeat
22 Refers to the passage of oxygenated blood through body tissues
23 Local venous inflammation
24 Sub normal body temperature
25 The primary medical problem is called the *presenting* _____
29 Necrotic layers that slough off

9 Anesthesia and Surgical Assisting

LEARNING OBJECTIVES

After reviewing this chapter, the reader will be able to:

- Describe and explain surgical terminology.
- Discuss principles of aseptic technique.
- Give examples of methods used to disinfect or sterilize surgical instruments and supplies.
- Describe procedures for preparing the surgical site and surgical team.
- Identify surgical instruments and explain their uses and maintenance.
- Compare and contrast types of suture needles and suture materials.
- Define the role of veterinary technicians in anesthesia and perioperative pain management.
- Describe the equipment used for anesthetizing animals.
- Prepare and maintain anesthetic machines and the associated equipment.
- List and describe the steps involved in anesthetizing animals for induction.
- Explain the procedures used in medicating and monitoring animals before, during, and after anesthesia.
- Prepare a small animal patient, anesthetic equipment, anesthetic agents, and accessories for general anesthesia.

SHORT ANSWER

1. After what length of time are skin sutures typically removed?

   _____

2. Other than sutures, what might be used for vessel ligation during surgery?

   _____

3. What is the most common form of gas sterilization found in the veterinary hospital, and for what equipment is it typically used?

   _____

   _____

4. Name these scissors in order from left to right.

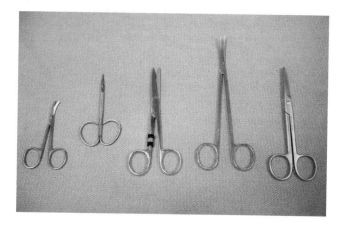

_____

_____

5. Name these forceps in order from left to right.

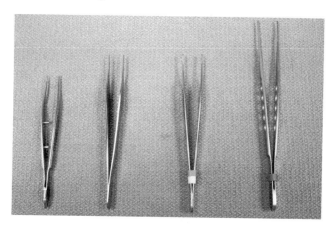

_____

_____

6. Why should hair be clipped liberally around the proposed surgical incision?

_____

7. Explain the major function of surgical masks.

_____

_____

8. What is the purpose of daily monitoring of body weight of a surgical patient?

_____

_____

9. Differentiate between contamination and infection of a wound.

_____

_____

10. List the steps in performing skin scrub on a patient.

_____

_____

_____

_____

_____

_____

11. Define *pain*.

_____

_____

12. Describe the proper method of folding a surgical gown.

_____

_____

_____

_____

_____

_____

13. List six of the physical signs of pain:

1. _____

2. _____

3. _____

4. _____

5. _____

6. _____

14. Describe the procedure for assisted gloving.

_____

_____

_____

_____

15. Why should an endotracheal tube be lubricated before insertion?

_____

_____

MATCHING—SURGICAL INSTRUMENTS

Match the following surgical instruments with their primary function.

1. _____ Hemostatic forceps   A. Used to incise tissue

2. _____ Needle holders   B. Used for cutting tissue

3. _____ Retractors   C. Grasp and manipulate curved needles

4. _____ Scissors   D. Clamp and hold tissue and blood vessels

5. _____ Scalpels and blades   E. Crushing instrument used to clamp blood vessels

6. _____ Tissue forceps   F. Used to retract tissue and improve exposure

MATCHING—SURGICAL PROCEDURES

Match the following surgical procedures with their definition.

1. _____ Herniorrhaphy   A. Incision into the intestine

2. _____ Orchiectomy   B. Removal of part or all of one or more mammary glands

3. _____ Gastrotomy   C. Incision into the urinary bladder

4. _____ Thoracotomy   D. Surgical removal of a claw

5. _____ Enterotomy   E. Incision into a simple stomach

6. _____ Cystotomy   F. Incision into the abdominal cavity

7. _____ Urethrotomy   G. Surgical removal of testes

8. _____ Laparotomy   H. Incision into thoracic cavity

9. _____ Mastectomy   I. Surgical repair of abnormal opening

10. _____ Onychectomy   J. Incision into the urethra

MATCHING—SURGICAL INCISIONS

Match the following surgical incisions with their location or benefit.

1. _____ Flank incision   A. Parallel to the last rib

2. _____ Ventral midline incision   B. Lateral and parallel to the ventral midline

3. _____ Median sternotomy   C. Perpendicular to long axis of body, caudal to last rib

4. _____ Paramedian incision   D. Offers excellent exposure of entire abdominal cavity

5. _____ Paracostal incision   E. Used when all lung fields need to be visualized

FILL IN THE BLANK

1. _____ is the term used to describe all precautions taken to prevent contamination or infection of a surgical wound.

2. Surgical procedures are described using _____ combined with root words.

3. _____ refers to the destruction of all microorganisms (bacteria, viruses, spores) on a surface or object.

4. Hospital-acquired infections are called _____.

5. Surgical mesh may be used to _____ or reinforce traumatized or devitalized tissues.

     Chapter **9** **Anesthesia and Surgical Assisting**

6. The unit used to create an environment of high-temperature, pressurized steam for sterilization of surgical instruments is called an _____.

7. _____ scissors have a blunt tip that, when introduced under the bandage edge, reduces the risk of cutting the underlying skin.

8. Organic nonabsorbable suture is available made of _____ or _____.

9. Surgical instrument manufacturers may recommend rinsing, cleaning, and sterilizing instruments in _____, because tap water contains minerals that cause discoloration and staining.

10. Surgical packs may not be completely sterilized if they are _____ or improperly loaded in the autoclave or gas sterilizer container.

11. Subcutaneous infections frequently progress to _____.

12. Before sterilization, surgical drapes are folded so that the _____ can be properly positioned over the surgical site without contaminating the drape.

13. A _____ should be available to place needed supplies and equipment on the instrument table or Mayo stand in an operating room.

14. _____ needles have a sharp tip that pierces and spreads tissues without cutting them.

15. Sterile preparation of the surgical site begins after transportation and _____ of the animal on the operating table.

16. The _____ area is used for storage of surgical supplies.

17. It is very helpful to know the normal behavior of the _____ when assessing for pain.

18. It has been demonstrated that pain is more easily managed if analgesics are given _____ before a patient experiences pain.

19. Pain results from the stimulation of nerve endings called _____.

20. Standard practice is to withhold food for _____ to _____ hours and water for _____ to _____ hours before anesthetic induction.

21. In high-volume clinics, when several people are involved in patient evaluation and preparation, _____ should be completed before any anesthetic procedure is done to ensure that appropriate items are available, important health issues have been addressed, and all involved persons have been informed.

22. Procedures classified as "dirty" or nonsterile are usually performed in the _____ area.

23. The term _____ refers to the ability of an organism to cause disease.

24. When the sterility of an item is in question, always consider it _____.

25. The surgical scrub should begin at the intended incision and continue out in concentric circles to an area at least _____ inches larger than the expected size of the sterile field needed.

26. The recommended method for verification of proper autoclave operation in veterinary clinics is _____.

27. A _____ is a monitoring device used to detect changes in oxygen saturation.

28. The correct relationship among _____, _____, and _____ is critical to destroy all living microorganisms.

29. Before they are autoclaved, instruments with box locks and hinges should be lubricated with _____ or _____.

30. Autoclaved instruments that have been placed in paper or plastic peel-back pouches and heat-sealed can be stored for _____.

SHORT ANSWER

1. Identify the three basic components of a suture needle:

   1. _____
   2. _____
   3. _____

2. What are five possible causes of wound dehiscence?

   1. _____
   2. _____
   3. _____
   4. _____
   5. _____

3. List the four main sources of potential contamination during surgery:

   1. _____
   2. _____
   3. _____
   4. _____

4. The four groups of nonabsorbable suture materials are:

   1. _____
   2. _____
   3. _____
   4. _____

5. List six pieces of surgical attire:

   1. _____
   2. _____
   3. _____
   4. _____
   5. _____
   6. _____

6. Name four indicators of infection after surgery:

    1. _____

    2. _____

    3. _____

    4. _____

7. Name seven factors that influence the effectiveness of all microbial control methods:

    1. _____

    2. _____

    3. _____

    4. _____

    5. _____

    6. _____

    7. _____

8. List at least three potential postoperative complications.

    _____

    _____

9. Explain why it is so important to use a monitoring chart and to be diligent in monitoring a patient.

    _____

    _____

    _____

    _____

10. Describe how to monitor respiration during an anesthetic procedure.

    _____

    _____

    _____

    _____

    _____

11. Describe how to monitor the cardiovascular function during an anesthetic procedure.

    _____

    _____

    _____

    _____

12. Describe what each of the following monitoring devices tell you about the patient.

Monitoring Device	Overview
Stethoscope	
Esophageal stethoscope	
Electrocardiograph	
Pulse oximeter	
Apnea monitor	
Doppler ultrasound	
Oscillometric method	
Capnometer	
Central venous pressure	

1. What gloving method is seen in the following figure? _____

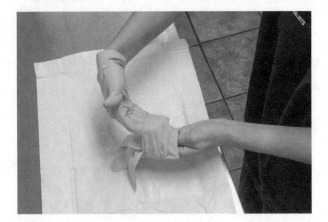

2. What procedure is pictured in the following figure? _____

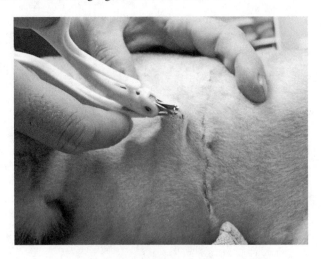

3. What sterilization equipment is seen in the following figure? _____

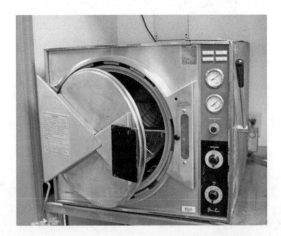

4. Examples of what type of suture are seen in the following figure? _____

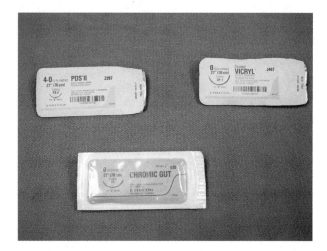

5. Identify both types of sterilization indicator tape seen in the following figure:

_____

_____

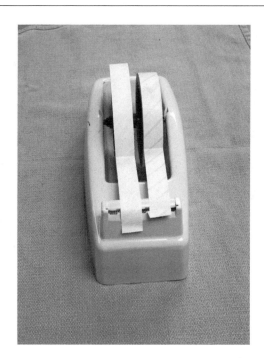

6. What surgical instruments are pictured in the following figure?

_____

_____

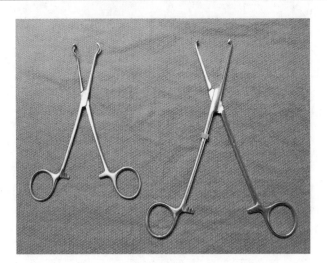

7. What procedure is seen in the following figure? _____

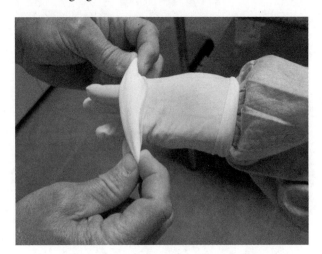

Fill in the blanks, and then find the terms in the word search below.

1. Infection in the abdominal cavity _____

2. Instruments designed to cut and remove bone pieces _____

3. The presence of microorganisms within or on an object or wound _____

4. Incision into the abdominal cavity; also called *celiotomy* _____

5. Large crushing instruments used to clamp blood vessels _____

6. Incision into the rumen _____

7. Incision into the thorax _____

8. Surgical removal of the lateral wall of the vertical portion of the external ear canal _____

9. Destruction of most living pathogenic microorganisms on animate (living) objects _____

10. Incision into the abdominal cavity; also called *laparotomy* _____

11. Instrument designed to bore holes in bone _____

12. Destruction of most pathogenic microorganisms on inanimate objects _____

13. Instrument designed to cut or shape bone and cartilage _____

14. Suture needles used in accessible places where the needle can be manipulated directly with the fingers

    _____

15. Incision into the urethra _____

16. Delicate scissors designed for fine, precise cuts, often used in ophthalmic procedures _____

17. A sterilization unit that creates high-temperature pressurized steam _____

18. Any strand of material that is used to approximate tissues or ligate blood vessels _____

19. Destruction of all microorganisms (bacteria, viruses, spores) on a surface or object _____

20. Use of a cauterizing needle tip or scalpel generating heat in tissue with a high-frequency current, to provide

    hemostasis in vessels less than 2 mm _____

21. Self-retaining retractor with a set screw to maintain tension on tissues, commonly used to retract abdominal wall

    _____

22. Instrument used to shape bone and cartilage _____

23. Instruments used to scrape surfaces of dense tissue _____

24. Incision into the stomach _____

25. Tissue scissors designed for cutting heavy tissue such as fascia _____

26. Surgical removal of part or all of one or more mammary glands _____

27. Self-retaining retractor with a box lock to maintain tension on tissues, commonly used in orthopedic surgeries

    _____

28. Delicate scissors designed for cutting fine, thin tissue _____

29. Condition in which microorganisms in the body or a wound multiply and cause harmful effects _____

30. Incision oriented perpendicular to the long axis of the body, caudal to the last rib _____

31. Protrude; refers to protrusion of an organ (viscera) through an incision _____

32. Incision into the intestine _____

```
L  A  S  N  T  N  O  I  T  A  Z  I  L  I  R  E  T  S  A  C  H  I  S  E  L
A  B  E  C  C  P  L  M  E  I  C  V  W  M  K  O  U  L  P  D  E  R  T  N  M
P  D  F  N  O  I  S  I  C  N  I  K  N  A  L  F  P  S  R  U  E  G  N  O  R
A  W  I  M  N  O  L  B  A  L  F  O  U  R  R  E  T  R  A  C  T  O  R  B  I
R  P  A  U  T  O  C  L  A  V  E  Y  T  E  V  E  D  C  N  P  Y  T  K  M  C
O  L  M  Q  A  R  O  T  C  A  R  T  E  R  I  P  L  E  G  A  R  C  E  E  N
T  B  U  T  M  G  H  J  O  I  K  M  X  E  W  T  O  P  I  T  N  M  L  I  V
O  U  P  R  I  N  F  E  C  T  I  O  N  P  I  L  Q  W  O  E  K  L  E  O  S
M  R  N  I  N  S  E  L  D  E  E  N  T  H  G  I  A  R  T  S  L  U  C  T  R
Y  E  O  K  A  U  Y  S  U  T  U  R  E  K  L  O  M  N  R  A  J  K  T  D  O
C  T  I  S  T  D  M  G  R  S  R  O  S  S  I  C  S  S  I  R  I  Y  R  E  S
J  H  T  E  I  E  O  A  Y  O  P  E  U  A  B  P  E  I  B  A  M  E  O  G  S
A  R  C  B  O  M  T  S  H  P  S  M  R  T  S  E  T  T  E  R  U  C  C  A  I
G  O  E  I  N  O  O  T  T  A  I  S  K  G  F  D  A  I  S  I  O  M  O  S  C
R  T  F  R  P  T  C  R  E  W  X  S  I  V  Z  J  Y  P  N  K  L  I  A  T  S
E  H  N  T  L  O  A  O  S  Y  W  I  B  C  E  L  I  O  T  O  M  Y  G  R  M
T  O  I  O  K  E  R  T  M  B  R  S  T  M  S  Q  D  B  L  U  P  T  U  O  U
A  M  S  I  E  T  O  O  Q  U  S  P  A  E  I  O  N  I  F  E  K  E  L  T  A
R  Y  I  G  I  S  H  M  A  S  T  E  C  T  O  M  Y  C  R  N  U  Y  A  O  B
E  J  D  N  S  O  T  Y  V  I  L  S  A  S  T  O  E  A  M  I  H  T  T  M  N
C  P  P  A  R  F  A  O  R  T  J  I  E  P  W  D  V  B  M  H  F  R  I  Y  E
S  D  I  E  N  C  P  L  A  S  I  T  I  N  O  T  I  R  E  P  W  D  O  L  Z
I  G  T  P  J  O  L  R  U  M  E  N  O  T  O  M  Y  S  K  E  I  P  N  I  T
V  N  R  L  M  L  O  T  M  T  P  A  Y  M  O  T  O  C  A  R  O  H  T  F  E
E  J  S  N  O  I  T  C  E  S  E  R  R  A  E  L  A  R  E  T  A  L  K  G  M
```

WORD SEARCH 2

Fill in the blanks, and then find the words in the word search below.

1. A mild to profound degree of CNS depression in which the patient is drowsy but may be aroused by painful

   stimuli _____

2. A chemical substance that can combine with a cell receptor and cause a reaction or create an active site

   _____

3. The narrowing of the blood vessels resulting from contraction of the muscular wall of the vessels, particularly the

   large arteries, small arterioles, and veins _____

4. A pressure gauge for comparing pressures of a gas _____

5. Frequency of breathing multiplied by the volume of each breath; it maintains normal concentrations of oxygen and carbon dioxide in the alveolar gas and, through the process of diffusion, also maintains normal partial pressures of oxygen and carbon dioxide in the blood flowing from the capillaries _____

6. The inability to feel pain while still conscious _____

7. A drug that produces numbness or stupor _____

8. A device used to measure blood pressure _____

9. Loss of feeling or awareness _____

10. The neural processes of encoding and processing noxious stimuli _____

11. The pressure of blood in the artery when the heart contracts _____

12. A drug or other chemical substance capable of reducing the physiologic activity of another chemical substance

_____

13. A measuring instrument that measures the oxygen in arterial blood _____

14. The action of certain medications that inhibits the transmission of parasympathetic nerve impulses and thereby

reduces spasms of smooth muscle (such as that, for example, in the bladder) _____

15. An unpleasant sensory or emotional experience associated with actual or potential tissue damage _____

16. Transient cessation of respiration _____

17. The rate at which the heart beats _____

18. Any disturbance of the heart's rhythm resulting in fewer-than-normal heart beats _____

19. The transport of oxygen from the outside air to the cells within tissues, and the transport of carbon dioxide in the

opposite direction _____

20. Excessive slowness in the action of the heart _____

21. An instrument used to measure the carbon dioxide (CO_2) concentration in an air sample _____

22. Pressure of blood in the artery when the heart relaxes between beats _____

23. Type of ultrasound device that a technician may use to sense the presence or absence of flow in blood vessels

_____

24. Abnormally rapid beating of the heart _____

25. Kind of stethoscope placed during anesthesia at the level of the heart to amplify the heart beat so that it is audible

from a distance _____

26. The lung volume representing the normal volume of air displaced between normal inspiration and expiration when

extra effort is not applied _____

27. Part of the anesthetic machine that receives medical gases from the pressure regulator _____

28. A common laboratory method of quantitative chemical analysis _____

29. Too much carbon dioxide in the blood is known as hypercarbia or _____

30. A state of relaxation and calmness characterized by a lack of anxiety or concern without significant drowsiness

_____

31. A medical instrument that is used to obtain a view of the vocal folds and the glottis, which is the space between

the cords _____

Chapter **9** Anesthesia and Surgical Assisting

```
C B J R N J Z R X S N E G C J S H P V N R X N G F
F I B Q G A M E E Q S I E I P N X B O D Z F L L B
B L G V O I R D B O R U L H R P F I Q N P T Z B P
H R G R H A A C P K E T Y E R I T N G I W V C A M
Y Z A W E T D H O A Z G Z Q H A E O X E Q R R B A
P A Q D Y N A Z C T M X W D Z T I T R A T I O N I
E E N O Y G I K N O T T C I R T S N O C O S A V M
R T N T E C P L M P N C L G W D G O L N G K L X H
C O S A A B A A O O H I F Q V O B G V H Z P E W T
A X L I I G N R C H U L A R Y N G O S C O P E P Y
P I E Z N O O I D Q C Z Y I A N E S T H E S I A H
N M R C M O C N N I W I R H D B U U N R C R S R
I E D E R E G A I F A Y T Y T R P E O H V A E E R
A T T L P W R A X S L P C N V H A I W R S P L M A
E E A T E T L P L H T I L I A H T C E R P N P U Y
R R I N O I T A R I P S E R L A R T Y R Y O P L D
B O C I L O T S Y S A O N Q L O E N S H T G O O A
N E P Y A O W Y P E H V Z I A M T N T T C R D V R
O S Z Q I N P D N C R Y T Q O C E S O X G A E L B
P U L S E Q W P D H F N O N W Y M P A U O P T A F
A I S E G L A N A H E A A K Z B W Q A I Z H I D E
B U E F M W V L J V X M D U V F O L K I D O M I G
E Y O U S G G B J K T X T P F Q L J N J N Q J T R
O I W X C I E F S A O X K D C V F G U T C X R X T
Z K U Y Y J R E X Q R A C D J V H A J V P Q F L L
```

Chapter **9** **Anesthesia and Surgical Assisting**

CROSSWORD

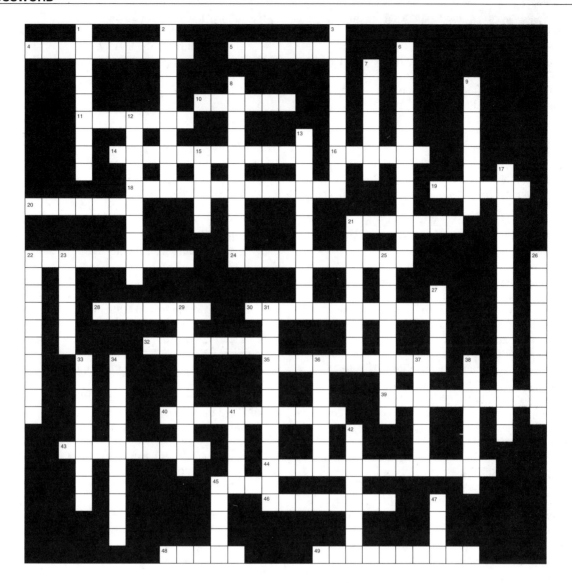

Across

4 The type of needle holders with a ratchet lock just distal to the thumb

5 The self-retaining retractor with a set screw to maintain tension on tissues, commonly used to retract abdominal wall

10 An instrument used to shape bone and cartilage

11 Type of suture needle with a sharp tip that pierces and spreads tissues without cutting them

14 Destruction of most pathogenic microorganisms on inanimate objects

16 Any strand of material that is used to approximate tissues or ligate blood vessels

18 The presence of microorganisms within or on an object or wound

19 The type of suture that is an organic nonabsorbable suture material with less tissue reaction than silk but that supports bacterial growth

20 Scissors with a blunt tip that can safely be introduced under a dressing for removal

21 The type of technique whereby all precautions are taken to prevent contamination and ultimately infection of a surgical wound

22 Incision into the stomach

24 Surgical removal of the testicles

28 A __ needle is a suture needle with two or three opposing sharp edges, used in tissues that are difficult to penetrate (7)

32 A __ section is the surgical removal of newborns via an abdominal incision

35 Surgical removal of a claw

39 The type of delicate scissors designed for cutting fine, thin tissue (10)

43 Type of needle holders with a ratchet lock just distal to the thumb, with a blade for cutting suture material

44 The process of heating a needle tip or scalpel before it is applied to tissue to provide hemostasis in vessels less than 2 mm in diameter

45 Another name for a rake retractor is the __ retractor

46 An instrument designed to bore holes in bone

48 Type of self-retaining retractor with a box lock to maintain tension on tissues, commonly used in orthopedic surgeries

49 Destruction of most living pathogenic microorganisms on animate objects

Down

1 Another name for a laparotomy

2 A __ incision is located lateral and parallel to the ventral midline of the animal

3 The tissue forceps with small serrations on the tips that cause minimal trauma but hold tissue securely

6 Surgical repair of a hernia by suturing the abnormal opening closed

7 An instrument used to scrape surfaces of dense tissue

8 Type of self-retaining retractor with a set screw to maintain tension on tissues; commonly used to retract the thoracic wall

9 Type of small hemostatic forceps with transverse jaw serrations

12 Protrude; refers to protrusion of an organ through an incision

13 Large crushing instruments used to clamp blood vessels

15 An incision oriented perpendicular to the long axis of the body, caudal to the last rib

17 Large crushing forceps often used to control large tissue bundles

21 A sterilization unit that creates high-temperature pressurized steam

22 Surgical fixation of the stomach to the abdominal wall

23 __ needles are suture needles that are joined with suture into a continuous unit

25 Surgical removal of part or all of one or more mammary glands

26 Incision into the intestine

27 Type of hemostatic forceps with transverse serrations that extend over only the distal portion of the jaws

29 Type of infection that is hospital acquired

31 Type of suture made of a single strand of material

33 A __ retractor is a self-retaining retractor with a box lock to maintain tension on tissues; commonly used in neurologic surgeries

34 Type of needle holders with a spring and latch mechanism for locking

36 Type of surgical gut that has been exposed to chrome or aldehyde to slow absorption

37 Type of needle holders with a ratchet lock at the proximal end of the handles of the holder, permitting locking and unlocking simply with a progressive squeezing of the instrument

38 Instruments designed to cut and remove bone pieces

41 Type of hemostatic forceps with transverse serrations that extend the entire jaw length

42 Keith or __ needles are used in accessible places where the needle can be manipulated directly with the fingers

45 Plain surgical gut is suture material made from the submucosa of __ intestine or serosa of bovine intestine

47 The type of delicate scissors designed for fine, precise cuts, often used in ophthalmic procedures

10 Laboratory Procedures

LEARNING OBJECTIVES

After reviewing this chapter, the reader will be able to:

- Describe methods used to collect samples for laboratory examination.
- Describe preparation of diagnostic samples for laboratory examination.
- List and describe common procedures used for hematologic examinations.
- List and describe methods for evaluation of hemostasis in dogs and cats.
- List and describe equipment needed for clinical chemistry and serology testing.
- List and describe the types of tests used in clinical chemistry testing.
- List the biochemical assays commonly performed to asses liver, kidney, and pancreatic function.
- List the types of immunologic tests.
- Discuss methods used to verify accuracy of laboratory test results.
- List and describe methods used to collect samples of body tissues and fluids for laboratory examination.
- List and describe microbiologic tests commonly performed to identify bacterial and fungal pathogens.
- List tests commonly performed in analyzing urine specimens.
- List common internal parasites of dogs and cats.
- List common external parasites of dogs and cats.

DEFINITIONS

Define the following terms:

1. Ocular lens _____

2. Anemia _____

3. Substage condenser _____

4. Centrifuge _____

5. Lipemia _____

6. Refractometer _____

7. Spectrophotometer _____

8. Lyophilized reagent _____

9. Impedance method _____

10. Control _____

11. Standard _____

12. Titer _____

13. Precision _____

14. Hemolysis _____

15. Packed cell volume _____

MATCHING—TERMS

1. _____ Photosensitive reagent
2. _____ Coombs test
3. _____ Study of microbes
4. _____ Immunochromatography
5. _____ Bacilli
6. _____ Cocci
7. _____ Microhematocrit
8. _____ Jaundice
9. _____ Study of fungi
10. _____ Indicates active infection

A. Icterus
B. Rapid immunomigration
C. Microbiology
D. Packed cell volume
E. Mycology
F. Chromogen
G. Rising antibody titer
H. Round-shaped bacteria
I. Rod-shaped bacteria
J. Detects autoantibodies

MATCHING—MICROBIOLOGY

1. _____ Fungi
2. _____ Multiple media in a single plate
3. _____ Thioglycollate
4. _____ Mueller-Hinton

A. Broth media
B. Bullseye
C. Dermatophyte test media
D. Culture and sensitivity

COMPLETE THE CHART

Culture	Description	Example
Selective		MacConkey EMB
	Contains specific growth factors for bacteria with strict nutrient requirements	
Differential		

SHORT ANSWER AND FILL IN THE BLANK

1. Differentiate among accuracy, precision, and reliability.

_____

_____

2. How would you prepare a 1:10 dilution of a patient sample?

_____

_____

_____

3. Define the following acronyms and the organs/tissues with which they are associated:

AST _____

ALT _____

ALP _____

BUN _____

4. List at least four tests used to evaluate the endocrine pancreas:

1. _____

2. _____

3. _____

4. _____

5. List the most common causes of false results on immunology tests.

_____

_____

_____

6. Describe instrument care and maintenance for chemistry analyzers.

_____

_____

_____

_____

7. Name the type of immunologic test that is most commonly used in veterinary practice.

_____

_____

8. List three methods of sample collection for microbiology:

1. _____

2. _____

3. _____

9. What is the most common cause of diagnostic failure with microbiology samples?

_____

_____

10. How should samples from animals with suspected zoonoses be submitted?

_____

_____

11. What reagent should be used to prepare a solid tissue sample for fungal testing?

_____

_____

12. Name two types of dermatophyte test media:

1. _____

2. _____

13. Name the media broth that is commonly used for urine cultures.

_____

14. Name the two most common uses of agglutination tests in small animal veterinary practice:

1. _____

2. _____

15. Of impression and scraping, which sample collection technique yields more cells?

_____

16. What type of collection technique is preferred for fistulated lesions?

_____

17. List the tests included in the CBC:

a. _____

b. _____

c. _____

d. _____

e. _____

f. _____

g. _____

h. _____

i. _____

j. _____

18. The PCV is also known as the _____.

19. List the four pieces of equipment needed to complete a CBC:

1. _____

2. _____

3. _____

4. _____

20. List at least four aspects to evaluate the quality of an Internet site:

 1. _____

 2. _____

 3. _____

 4. _____

21. List four commonly used histology fixatives:

 1. _____

 2. _____

 3. _____

 4. _____

22. List three items considered internal laboratory records:

 1. _____

 2. _____

 3. _____

23. Describe the contents of a laboratory SOP.

 _____

 _____

 _____

24. Describe preparation of a patient for blood collection.

 _____

 _____

25. List four methods of urine collection:

 1. _____

 2. _____

 3. _____

 4. _____

26. Gross examination of urine should include evaluation of color, _____, _____, and

 _____.

27. List the four components of the complete urinalysis:

 1. _____

 2. _____

 3. _____

 4. _____

28. Samples collected before an animal has eaten are referred to as _____. Samples collected after an animal has eaten are referred to as _____.

29. List the steps for using the refractometer:

    1. _____

    2. _____

    3. _____

    4. _____

    5. _____

    6. _____

30. _____ is the preferred anticoagulant for hematology testing.

31. Flea larvae feed on _____ _____.

32. Organisms in the phylum Arthropoda are characterized by the presence of _____ _____.

33. Parasites residing on the surface of the host are called _____.

34. Life cycle of nematodes follows a standard pattern of developmental stages. Name them:

    1. _____

    2. _____

    3. _____

35. Arachnids include:

    1. _____

    2. _____

    3. _____

    4. _____

36. Name the two main classifications of ticks:

    1. _____

    2. _____

37. Name the two main classifications of mites:

    1. _____

    2. _____

38. Describe the method used to recover ova of tapeworms.

    _____

    _____

    _____

39. Name materials needed for a direct smear:

1. _____

2. _____

3. _____

4. _____

FILL IN THE BLANK

1. In the veterinary practice laboratory, sensitive equipment such as chemistry analyzers and cell counters must be physically separated from _____ and water baths.

2. High-quality Internet sites are _____ with no vested interest in the content.

3. The _____ mandates specific laboratory practices that must be incorporated into the laboratory safety policy.

4. Concentrations of dilutions are usually expressed as ratios of the _____ volume to the new volume.

5. When viewed through a compound light microscope, an object appears _____ and reversed.

6. Excess oil on microscope lenses may require the use of _____ for cleaning.

7. A horizontal centrifuge head, also known as the _____ type, has specimen cups that hang vertically when the centrifuge is at rest.

8. The microhematocrit centrifuge is configured to accommodate _____ tubes.

9. The most common uses of the refractometer are determination of the _____ of urine or other fluids and the _____ concentration of plasma or other fluids.

10. The refractometer is calibrated with _____.

11. All spectrophotometers contain a light source, prism, _____, photodetector, and readout device.

12. _____ _____ are calibrated to count cells in specified size ranges.

13. Before processing, refrigerated blood samples must be _____.

14. For many hematology analyzers, _____ _____ are periodically performed to make sure that the diluting solution is not contaminated and/or the glassware and tubing are not dirty.

15. A small dish of _____ may be placed inside an incubator to maintain proper humidity.

TRUE OR FALSE

1. _____ Samples for hematology testing should be collected from a properly fasted animal.

2. _____ The cephalic vein is the preferred site for large quantities of blood collection in all dogs and cats.

3. _____ Heparin is the preferred anticoagulant for hematology testing.

4. _____ Sodium citrate anticoagulant is used for coagulation tests.

5. _____ Impedance analyzers quantify cells in a sample based on their size and density.

6. _____ The veterinary clinical laboratory should be located in an area that is separate from other hospital operations.

7. _____ Drafts can carry dust, which may contaminate specimens and interfere with test results.

8. _____ For long-term storage of fluid samples (e.g., serum, plasma), a chest freezer or freezer that is self-defrosting should be used.

9. _____ Laboratory safety policies are mandated by the U.S. Department of Agriculture.

10. _____ The ratios ½ = 1 : 2 = 0.5 all designate the same concentration.

11. _____ To prepare a 1 : 10 dilution of a patient sample, combine 10 microliters (µL) of sample with 10 µL of distilled water.

12. _____ Samples that are hemolyzed, icteric, or lipemic may yield inaccurate results with many of the automated analyzers.

13. _____ If a standard solution of bilirubin contains 20 mg/dL and is diluted 1 : 10, the concentration of the dilution would then be 1 mg/dL.

14. _____ Liver function tests referred to as the leakage enzyme tests include AST, ALT, and ALP.

15. _____ Total serum protein concentrations include all plasma proteins except fibrinogen and certain other coagulation proteins.

16. _____ Dehydrated animals usually have elevated total protein values.

17. _____ Dehydration can lead to azotemia.

18. _____ Aseptic technique is critical when collecting microbiology samples.

19. _____ Formalin fumes can render samples unsatisfactory for analysis.

20. _____ Carbon dioxide released by dry ice may kill bacteria and viruses.

21. _____ Microbiology samples collected after medical treatment has started produce better results.

22. _____ Some cytology samples require centrifugation in order to concentrate cells.

23. _____ For impression smears from active lesions, an initial impression should not be made until after the lesion has been cleaned.

24. _____ All fine-needle aspirate sites should be surgically prepped before sample collection.

25. _____ Soft tissue masses require large-bore needles for aspiration.

26. _____ Longer fixative times improve staining quality and do not harm cytology samples.

27. _____ Vaginal cytology samples are collected with the animal in a standing position, with the tail elevated.

28. _____ It is not necessary to clean the external genitalia prior to obtaining a vaginal cytology sample.

29. _____ Most histologic fixatives are capable of penetrating 2 to 4 mm in 24 hours.

30. _____ Histology samples are usually collected by biopsy.

31. _____ The most concentrated urine sample is one collected after exercise.

32. _____ If refrigerated, urine samples should be warmed to body temperature before analysis.

33. _____ Urine dipstick analysis should be performed on well-mixed, room temperature, and chemically preserved urine.

34. _____ Containers of urine dipsticks must be stored in the refrigerator.

35. _____ Abdominocentesis does not require surgical preparation. Thoracentesis does require surgical preparation.

36. _____ The organism that a parasite lives in or on is called its host.

37. _____ Nematodes are commonly called roundworms because of their cylindrical body shape.

38. _____ Some adult flies glue their eggs to the hairs of the host.

39. _____ Most mite infestations are transmitted by indirect contact with an infested animal.

40. _____ An object viewed under the 40× objective through a 10× ocular lens is 400 times larger in diameter than the unmagnified object.

104

LISTS AND SHORT ANSWER

1. List six zoonotic internal parasites:

   1. _____

   2. _____

   3. _____

   4. _____

   5. _____

   6. _____

2. List the six electrolytes that are most commonly measured in the veterinary practice lab:

   1. _____

   2. _____

   3. _____

   4. _____

   5. _____

   6. _____

MULTIPLE CHOICE

1. When doing a fecal smear, it should be:
   a. thick.
   b. thin.
   c. watery.
   d. dry.

2. To prepare a fecal sample for centrifugation, you should use:
   a. 3 to 6 g of feces.
   b. 2 to 5 g of feces.
   c. quarter-size amount.
   d. half-dollar–size amount.

3. Tests of kidney function include:
   a. AST and ALT.
   b. fructosamine and glucose.
   c. amylase and lipase.
   d. urea nitrogen and creatinine.

4. Red-tinged plasma is referred to as:
   a. hemolyzed.
   b. icteric.
   c. lipemic.
   d. normal.

5. Yellow-tinged plasma is referred to as:
   a. hemolyzed.
   b. icteric.
   c. lipemic.
   d. normal.

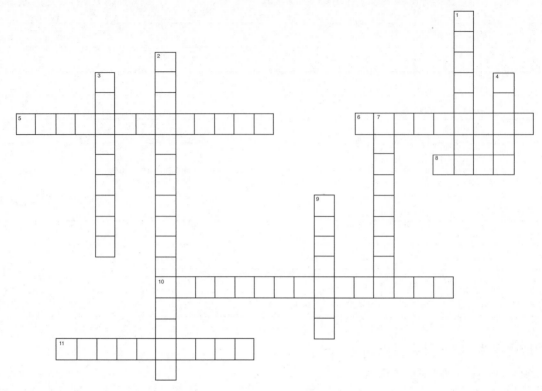

Across

5 Instrument used to measure the refractive index of a solution
6 bleeding from the nares
8 preferred anticoagulant for hematology
10 includes maternal antibodies from colostrum
11 Instrument used to separate substances of different densities that are in a solution

Down

1 nonbiologic solution of an analyte, usually in distilled water, with a known concentration
2 decreased number of platelets
3 thrombocytes
4 the most common type of immunologic tests performed in veterinary clinics
7 The magnitude of random errors and the reproducibility of measurements
9 Presence of fatty material in plasma or serum

11 Diagnostic Imaging

LEARNING OBJECTIVES

After reviewing this chapter, the reader will be able to:

- Describe the components of the x-ray machine and the function of each part.
- Explain how x-rays are produced.
- Discuss the factors that affect radiographic quality.
- Describe techniques and devices used to optimize radiographic quality.
- Discuss the dangers of radiation and methods to avoid radiation injury.
- Describe the procedures used to develop radiographs.
- Explain proper positioning of animals for various radiographic studies.
- Describe the basic physics of ultrasound.
- List the components of ultrasound machines and the function of each part.
- List the non–x-ray imaging modalities, and provide an overview of each.

FILL IN THE BLANK OR CIRCLE THE BEST ANSWER

1. Radiographs that show a **long** or **short** (circle one) scale of contrast have a few black and white shades, with a **few** or **many** (circle one) shades of gray. A **long** or **short** (circle one) scale of contrast has black-and-white shades, with a **few** or **many** (circle one) shades of gray in between. For most studies, a **short** or **long** (circle one) scale of contrast is desirable.

2. What four factors affect the proper scale of radiographic contrast?

   1. _____

   2. _____

   3. _____

   4. _____

3. Denser tissues, such as bone, absorb **greater** or **lesser** (circle one) amounts of x-rays and appear **white** or **black** (circle one) on a radiograph, whereas less dense tissues, such as lung tissue, absorb **greater** or **lesser** (circle one) amounts of x-rays and appear **white** or **black** (circle one) on the finished radiograph.

4. As kVp **increases** or **decreases** (circle one), the scale of contrast gets longer and there is **more** or **less** (circle one) exposure latitude, which is forgiving of minor technique errors.

5. The National Council on Radiation Protection and Measurements recommends that the dose for occupationally

   exposed persons not exceed _____ per year. The MPD for nonoccupational persons is _____ %

   of the dose for occupationally exposed persons, or _____ per year. This is known as the

   _____. Also, a fetus should not receive more than _____ during the entire gestational

   period.

6. Calculate the remaining value:

   a. 100 mA and $\frac{1}{20}$ sec: _____ mAs

   b. 300 mA and 5 mAs: _____ sec

   c. 10 mAs and $\frac{1}{25}$ sec _____ mA

7. In order to achieve optimal ultrasound imaging, what preparations are involved?

   1. _____

   2. _____

   3. _____

   4. _____

   5. _____

8. What fasting procedures are required for preparation for endoscopy?

   _____

9. Explain some procedures involved with the care of endoscopes:

   1. _____

   2. _____

   3. _____

   4. _____

   5. _____

   6. _____

   7. _____

   8. _____

   9. _____

   10. _____

   11. _____

10. List six potential causes of film fogging:

   1. _____

   2. _____

   3. _____

   4. _____

   5. _____

   6. _____

11. List important safety rules that should be kept in mind while exposing an x-ray film:

   1. _____

   2. _____

   3. _____

   4. _____

   5. _____

   6. _____

   7. _____

   8. _____

12. Fill in the meanings of the acronyms and abbreviations:

   1. REM   _____

   2. SV   _____

   3. rad   _____

   4. FFD   _____

   5. ALARA   _____

   6. MPD   _____

   7. OFD   _____

COMPLETE THE CHART

Body Part	Cranial or Proximal Landmark	Caudal or Distal Landmark	Center Landmark	Comments
Abdomen				Take at peak _____
Thorax				Take at peak _____
Pelvis			✕	✕
Stifle				✕
Radius and ulna				✕
Lumbar vertebrae			✕	To increase detail _____

MATCHING

Match the imaging technique/substance with its purpose.

1. _____ Scintigraphy

2. _____ Tesla

3. _____ Computer tomography

4. _____ Fiberoptic endoscope

5. _____ Air

6. _____ Radioactive iodine

7. _____ Sodium diatrizoate

8. _____ Gadolinium

9. _____ Nonionic water-soluble iodides

10. _____ Barium

11. _____ Linear array

12. _____ Sector scan

A. Treatment for hyperthyroidism

B. MRI contrast media

C. Transmits images using glass fibers

D. Used for excretory urography

E. Measure of a magnetic field

F. Used for myelography

G. Nuclear medicine

H. Negative contrast media

I. Positive contrast agent for GI studies

J. Ultrasound transducer that produces pie-shaped image

K. Produces cross-sectional image

L. Ultrasound transducer that produces rectangular image

MATCHING—KEY TERMS

A. Terms Associated with Radiographic Quality

1. _____ Anode heel effect

2. _____ Radiographic density

3. _____ Radiographic contrast

4. _____ Subject density

5. _____ Radiographic detail

6. _____ Artifacts

7. _____ Penumbra

A. Loss of detail resulting from geometric lack of sharpness

B. Unwanted density in the form of blemishes

C. Sharp interfaces between tissues and organs

D. Unequal distribution of the x-ray beam intensity

E. Differences in radiographic density between adjacent areas on a radiographic image

F. Degree of blackness on a radiograph

G. Ability of the different tissue densities to absorb x-rays

B. Terms Associated with Processing

1. _____ Acidifier

2. _____ Activator

3. _____ Fixing agent

4. _____ Hardener

5. _____ Main purpose of the developer

6. _____ Main purpose of the fixer

7. _____ Preservative

8. _____ Reducing agent

9. _____ Restrainer

10. _____ Solvent

A. Causes film emulsion to swell

B. Found in both solutions; sodium or potassium sulfite is used

C. Prevents the reducing agents from affecting the unsensitized crystals

D. Provides an alkaline pH in the range of 9.8 to 11.4

E. Hardens and prevents excessive swelling of the film emulsion

F. Neutralizes any alkaline developer remaining on the film

G. Clears the unchanged silver halide crystals from the film emulsion, leaving the black metallic silver

H. Changes the sensitized silver halide crystals into black metallic silver

I. Converts the exposed silver halide crystals to black metallic silver

J. Sodium or ammonium thiosulfate that clears the remaining silver halide crystals in the fixer

C. Terms Associated with Positioning

1. _____ Ventral (V):

2. _____ Dorsal (D):

3. _____ Medial (M):

4. _____ Lateral (L):

5. _____ Cranial (Cr):

6. _____ Caudal (Cd):

7. _____ Rostral (R):

8. _____ Palmar (Pa):

9. _____ Plantar (Pl):

10. _____ Proximal (Pr):

11. _____ Distal (Di):

A. Situated closer to the point of attachment or origin

B. Situated on the caudal aspect of the rear limb, distal to the tarsus

C. Areas on the head situated toward the nose

D. Body area situated toward the median plane or midline

E. Situated away from the point of attachment or origin

F. Structures or areas situated toward the head

G. Body area situated toward the underside of quadrupeds

H. Structures or areas situated toward the tail

I. Situated on the caudal aspect of the front limb, distal to the carpus

J. Body area situated toward the back or topline of quadrupeds

K. Body area situated away from the median plane or midline

MULTIPLE CHOICE

1. What are the agents along with the solvent that are in the fixer?
   a. reducing agent, fixing agent, accelerator, and acidifier
   b. fixing agent, preservative, hardener, and acidifier
   c. reducing agent, accelerator, preservative, restrainer, and hardener
   d. buffer, accelerator, acidifier, clearing agent, and hardener

2. Unequal distribution of the x-ray beam results in the phenomenon referred to as:
   a. penumbra effect.
   b. heel effect.
   c. ALARA.
   d. hyperechoic.

3. The temperature of the manual developer is 65° F (18° C). If one were to process at this temperature, the time should be:
   a. 3¾ minutes.
   b. 5¾ minutes.
   c. 6¼ minutes.
   d. 7½ minutes.

4. You are doing a safelight quality control test with an initial moderate exposure. There is no area of increased density. This means that:
   a. there is no problem with the safelight or light leaking around the door.
   b. you need to get a brand-new safelight because you will always have fogging.
   c. you have less than 30 seconds to get the film in the processing solutions.
   d. you must have completed the test incorrectly.

5. Which of the following choices is ordered from lowest subject density to greatest subject density?
   a. metal, bone, water, fat, and gas
   b. fat, water, gas, bone, and metal
   c. water, gas, fat, bone, and metal
   d. gas, fat, water, bone, and metal

6. With regard to radiation exposure of pregnant women and those under 18:
   a. technically the law states that there is no more concern for these than for others who are occupationally exposed.
   b. the law states that they should never be in the room during the exposure.
   c. the dermis, bone, and blood cells are the most sensitive to ionizing radiation.
   d. the growth and gonadal cells are most sensitive to ionizing radiation.

7. The *quality of the beam* refers to:
   a. kVp.
   b. mAs.
   c. rectification that is required.
   d. darkness of the radiograph.

8. Scatter will be more noticeable if there is a thicker patient and:
   a. lower kVp and larger field size.
   b. lower kVp and smaller field size.
   c. higher kVp and smaller field size.
   d. higher kVp and larger field size.

9. The rare earth screens emit which color of light when they fluoresce?
   a. green
   b. blue
   c. clear
   d. mauve

10. If involved with MRI it is important to keep in mind that:
    a. latex gloves or lab coats are not needed if handling radionuclide or a radioactive patient.
    b. there is no excretion of radionuclides in urine and feces.
    c. isolation or a well-ventilated area is not required if radionuclides are injected.
    d. an anesthetic machine could cause serious damage to the MRI machine.

TRUE OR FALSE

1. _____ Penumbra can be minimized by increasing the size of the focal spot.

2. _____ If the limb is not parallel to the film, you may have foreshortening.

3. _____ The collimator in an x-ray tube head focuses the primary beam to a narrower image.

4. _____ For safety reasons, it is best to use a lower mA but a longer time in seconds.

5. _____ The higher the mA setting on the x-ray machine, the greater the number of x-rays produced. The higher the kVp, the greater the penetrating power of the x-rays.

6. _____ Keeping all other factors constant and changing the mAs from 5 to 10 will double the radiographic density.

7. _____ If there was no image on a film that was exposed to radiation and it was processed normally, the film would appear black.

8. _____ Light leakage around one edge of the film will appear white.

9. _____ Thumbnail pressure on a film after exposure but before processing will show as a crescent black mark.

10. _____ A hair on the film during exposure to radiation will appear black.

11. _____ Rare-earth phosphors are the most common blue-light–emitting phosphors.

12. _____ Digital radiography includes computed radiography (CR), digital radiography (DR), and coupled charged devices (CCD) technologies.

13. _____ For CCD digital radiography, the imaging plate (IP) contains a photostimulable phosphor.

14. _____ Digital radiographs, CT scans, MRI images, and ultrasound images are all stored using a universally accepted format known as DICOM.

15. _____ A PACS has the advantage of storing multiple patients' images and making images available to multiple computers within a hospital or a network of hospitals.

16. _____ With regard to x-ray gloves, radiation cannot penetrate lead gloves.

17. _____ Effects may be somatic or carcinogenic when radiation comes in contact with the cells of living tissue— passing through the cells with no effect, producing cell damage that is repairable or not repairable, or killing the cells.

18. _____ Tissues that are most sensitive to ionizing radiation are those with rapidly growing or reproducing cells including lymphocytic series, reproductive organs, GI tissues, and the lens of the eye.

19. _____ Intrauterine lethality is most critical from 0 to 9 days, while the period of organogenesis (10 days to 6 weeks) is associated with the greatest risk of congenital malformation in the fetus.

20. _____ To verify gloves and gowns are not damaged, obtain radiographs on them at 5 mAs and 80 kVp every 18 months.

21. _____ The most important feature of a darkroom is that it must be light tight.

22. _____ Radiographs must be labeled with the clinic name and location, the date the radiograph was taken, the owner's name, and the patient's name.

23. _____ A red lightbulb can substitute as a safelight filter.

24. _____ The safelight that is effective against blue-light–sensitive film can also be used with green-light–sensitive film.

25. _____ If either the replenishing method or the exhausted method is used for manual processing, the chemicals should be changed every 3 months.

26. _____ In automatic processors the chemicals are kept at temperatures around 80° F (27° C).

27. _____ Label the radiograph of the oblique so that a marker is placed to indicate the direction of entry and exit of the primary beam.

28. _____ It is essential in endoscopy that the endotracheal tube cuff remain uninflated during extubation.

29. _____ Microchips can cause serious damage to an MRI machine.

30. _____ Another term for nuclear medicine is scintigraphy, an imaging modality that uses radionuclides.

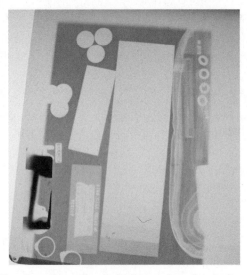

1. Why does the radiograph show a low density?

_____

_____

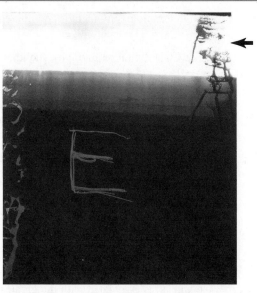

2. This film was exposed to light and then processed. Why would there be a clear area at the upper portion of the film? What has caused the blackened area under the arrow?

_____

_____

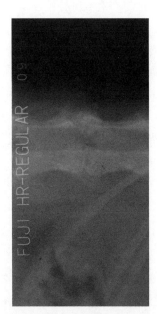

3. Is this a low- or high-contrast film?

_____

_____

4. Has this film been exposed to radiation? What has caused the darkened areas at the edges?

_____

_____

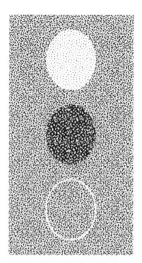

5. From upper to lower, what are the three ultrasound areas shown in the circled areas?

_____

_____

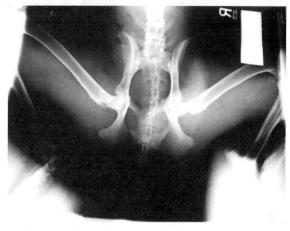

6. What are the white areas at the corners of the radiograph, and why is this a problem?

_____

_____

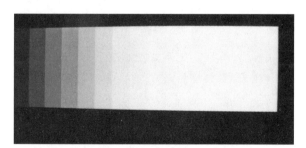

7. The whitest area is the thickest or thinnest portion of the step wedge?

_____

_____

8. From left to right, what tissue densities are represented with each area?

_____

_____

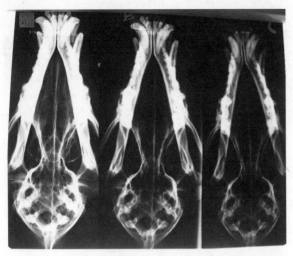

9. The skull on the left is larger because of increased or decreased OFD. Assuming that there has been a corresponding change in exposure factors, the skull on the left could also be larger because of a **shorter** or **longer** SID? (Choose one)

_____

_____

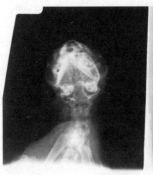
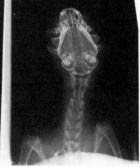

10. The skull on the left has lower or higher kVP and is considered to have **lower** or **higher** contrast? (Choose one)

_____

_____

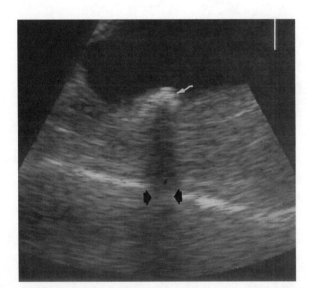

11. What artifact is shown? The white arrow is pointing to the _____, whereas the black arrows are pointing to the _____.

_____

_____

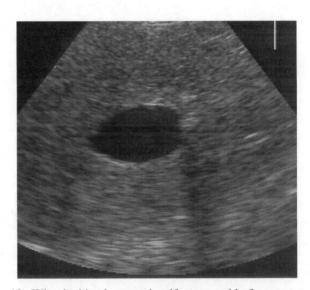

12. What is this ultrasound artifact caused by?

_____

_____

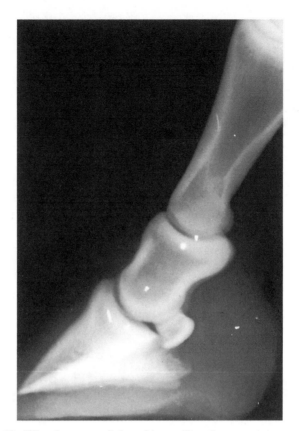

13. What has caused the white artifacts?

_____

_____

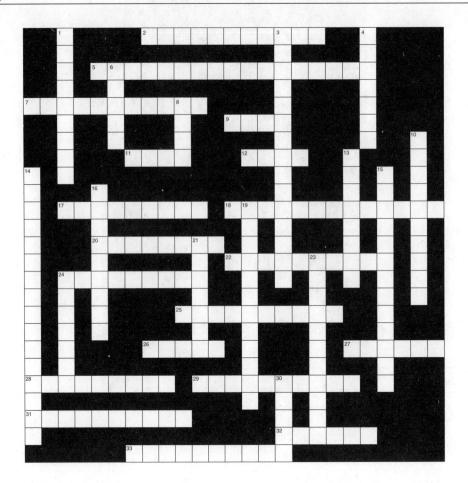

Across

2 An imaging technique using contrast media to visualize the spinal cord

5 MRI, or __ __ imaging, is a modality that uses a magnetic field that recognizes the natural resonance of the atoms within the body to produce images

7 The __ peak is the maximum voltage applied across an x-ray tube that determines the energy of the electrons produced

9 The acronym for dedicated computer systems that are used for storing, retrieval, transferring, and manipulating images

11 One form of electromagnetic radiation

12 A __ is a device that is made up of lead strips interspaced with a radiolucent material; it absorbs scatter radiation

17 Substances that emit light when exposed to electromagnetic radiation

18 The current produced by the x-ray tube during an exposure

20 A structure not normally present but visible on a radiograph; diminishes the quality of the radiograph

22 An example of when there is greater radiation intensity on the negatively charged side of an x-ray tube owing to the angle of the target on the positively charged side

24 A low-wattage lightbulb and special filter that will not affect radiographic film

25 A device on an x-ray machine that consists of lead plates and is used to reduce scatter radiation

26 A chemical solution that clears unchanged silver halide crystals on an exposed x-ray film

27 The __ image is the invisible image that is within the emulsion of an x-ray film produced after the film has been exposed to light

28 __ ___ elements are photosensitive elements such as lanthanum oxybromide and gadolinium oxysulfide that are in an x-ray–intensifying screen

29 The device on an ultrasound machine that emits and receives a sound wave signal that converts the waves into electrical impulses

31 Ultrasound is a modality that uses __ __ that interact with tissues interfaces and are reflected back to create an image

32 Negative contrast agents are gases such as __ and carbon dioxide that are radiolucent on radiographs and are used to outline organs

33 The ___ - ___ distance is the distance between the object being radiographed and the film or plate

Down

1 A chemical solution that converts exposed silver halide crystals to black metallic silver

3 Being able to store a latent image that may be freed as light when stimulated by a scanning laser

4 The dose of radiation equivalent to the absorbed dose by tissue

6 The positively charged electrode in an x-ray tube

8 The measured unit of radiation dose that is absorbed as a result of ionized radiation

10 CT, or computed __, is a modality that uses an x-ray tube that freely rotates around a patient, creating a dataset of images

13 __ radiography is a type of digital radiography that uses a cassette screen system

14 A type of medium such as barium or iodine that is radiopaque on radiographs used to visualize organs in the body

15 __ __ radiography is a type of digital radiography that uses an imaging plate of detectors connected directly to a computer system

16 The ___ -___ distance is the distance that is measured from the target of the x-ray tube to the radiographic film or plate

19 __ screens are plates within the x-ray cassette that are composed of phosphorescent crystals that function to emit light

21 The negatively charged electrode in an x-ray tube that produces electrons

23 An imaging technique that produces a continual stream of images

24 __ radiation is the radiation created as a result of the interaction of primary beam x-ray photons and body parts or matter that travel in a different direction and are composed of lower energies

30 The acronym for the universal method in which medical imaging can be stored and transferred

12 Avian and Exotic Animal Care and Nursing

LEARNING OBJECTIVES

After reviewing this chapter, the reader will be able to:

- State the general characteristics of mice, rats, hamsters, gerbils, guinea pigs, chinchillas, rabbits, and ferrets.
- Discuss husbandry and principles of sanitation for small mammals.
- Describe techniques for general nursing care of rodents, rabbits, and ferrets.
- Describe techniques used for diagnosing and treating disease in small mammals.
- Describe the unique features of the anatomy of birds and basic biology of common reptile species.
- Discuss the basic behavior of birds, reptiles, and amphibians.
- Discuss the basics of client education, husbandry, and nutrition for the avian, reptilian, and amphibian species.
- Describe how to obtain a complete and thorough history of avian, reptilian, and amphibian patients.
- Explain the different capture and restraint techniques used for birds, reptiles, and amphibians.
- Identify methods of sample collection for laboratory analysis.
- Describe how to obtain high-quality diagnostic images of avian, reptilian, and amphibian patients.
- Discuss nursing care and supportive therapy techniques for avian, reptilian, and amphibian patients.
- Identify and discuss some of the common diseases of avian, reptilian, and amphibian patients of the veterinary clinic.

LABELING—AVIAN RESPIRATORY SYSTEM

Identify the elements in this diagram of the avian respiratory system, lateral view.

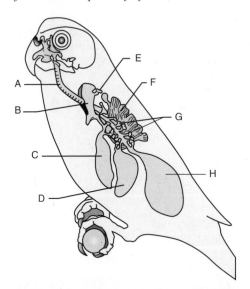

A. _____   E. _____

B. _____   F. _____

C. _____   G. _____

D. _____   H. _____

LABELING—FEATHERS

Identify the types of feathers shown.

A   B   C   D   E

A. _____   D. _____

B. _____   E. _____

C. _____

MATCHING

Match the avian terms with their definitions.

1. _____ Anisodactyl

2. _____ Coprodeum

3. _____ Pneumatized

4. _____ Coverts

5. _____ Proctodeum

6. _____ Keel

7. _____ Remiges

8. _____ Choana

9. _____ Urodeum

10. _____ Uropygial

11. _____ Zygodactyl

A. Caudal part of the cloaca

B. Cranial portion of the cloaca that receives feces from the rectum

C. Large sternum

D. Middle part of the cloaca

E. Another term for large primary flight feathers

F. Containing air

G. Arrangement of feet with second and third toes facing forward and first and fourth toes directed backward

H. Located dorsally at the base of the tail

I. Arrangement of feet so that three toes point forward and one toe points to the rear

J. Body feathers that provide surface coverage

K. Slitlike opening in the roof of the mouth

SHORT ANSWER, FILL IN THE BLANK, AND LISTS

1. What are some principles that should be kept in mind when feeding avians?

   1. _____
   2. _____
   3. _____
   4. _____
   5. _____

2. Signs of respiratory distress in a bird include the following:

   1. _____
   2. _____
   3. _____
   4. _____
   5. _____
   6. _____
   7. _____
   8. _____

3. List at least five potential causes of lower airway avian emergencies:

   1. _____
   2. _____
   3. _____
   4. _____
   5. _____

4. Signs of egg retention include:

   1. _____
   2. _____
   3. _____
   4. _____
   5. _____
   6. _____

5. What signs should you watch for when determining if a bandage needs to be changed?

   1. _____
   2. _____
   3. _____
   4. _____

6. Regarding sites for the administration of fluid and medication in lizards:

   1. When handling reptiles, wear latex or examination gloves to protect yourself from exposure to _____

   2. The most common routes are usually _____ and _____ sites.

   3. A _____ feeding tube is generally used when force feeding most reptile and amphibian species.

   4. A _____ feeding tube is generally used when force feeding most avian species.

   5. Chelonians, lizards, and snakes commonly present in emergency situations as a result of _____ injuries.

7. What are some ways to minimize dominance behavior problems in parrots?

   _____

   _____

   _____

   _____

   _____

   _____

   _____

8. List the common venipuncture sites for the following species:

   Chelonians _____

   Lizards _____

   Snakes _____

9. List the common intravenous catheter sites in reptiles:

   Chelonians _____

   Lizards _____

   Snakes _____

DEFINITIONS

Define the following terms:

1. diastema _____

2. Harderian gland _____

3. lagomorph _____

4. haustra _____

5. catabolic _____

MATCHING

Match the disease or conditions with the description.

1. _____ Bordetella bronchiseptica

2. _____ Canine distemper

3. _____ Coccidia

4. _____ Heat stroke

5. _____ Dysecdysis

6. _____ Pododermatitis

7. _____ *Mesocricetus auratus*

8. _____ West Nile virus

9. _____ Chlamydiosis

10. _____ Psoroptes

11. _____ Phototoxicity

12. _____ Pacheco disease

13. _____ Red leg

14. _____ Periodontal disease

A. Gum infection common in ferrets

B. Zoonotic disease that causes psittacosis in humans and avian chlamydiosis in avian species

C. Cutaneous bacterial infection

D. Rabbit ear mite

E. Common endoparasite in rabbits

F. Difficulty in shedding the skin in reptiles

G. Pressure necrosis of the plantar surface of the metatarsal area seen in obese rabbits

H. Herpetic virus seen in psittacids

I. Sensitivity light

J. Susceptibility in guinea pigs

K. Chinchillas prone to this with increased humidity

L. Mosquito-borne disease that primarily infects horses, humans, and birds

M. Golden hamster

N. Fatal disease of ferrets

TRUE OR FALSE

1. _____ The average adult bird has a core body temperature of 38° to 42.5° C (105° to 112° F).

2. _____ If a blood feather needs to be removed, it should be pulled in the direction opposite the direction in which the feather is growing.

3. _____ In flushing a wound in birds, care needs to be taken that the puncture is not communicating with an air sac.

4. _____ The uropygial gland is absent in the ostrich, emu, cassowary, bustard, and frogmouth and in many pigeons, woodpeckers, and Amazon parrots.

5. _____ Wing trimming should be done only on primary flight feathers.

6. _____ The proventriculus or true stomach is very similar to the stomach of mammals, containing digestive acid and enzymes.

7. _____ The largest muscles in the avian body are the pectorals.

8. _____ Grit is required in the gizzard for proper digestion of hard foods.

9. _____ When a bird is stressed, there is an increased fecal component to the droppings because the droppings pass before lower intestinal water resorption occurs.

10. _____ In most birds, ovulation to egg laying takes approximately 15 hours.

11. _____ The bird's circulatory system differs from that of mammals in that the red blood cells of birds are oval and contain a nucleus, but birds do have lymph nodes.

12. _____ To minimize behavior problems in cockatoos, it is best to repeatedly pet the bird over its back and tail.

13. _____ To properly capture birds, towels should be used as much as possible and gloves and bare hands should be discouraged.

14. _____ A good place to capture a bird is from the owner's shoulders.

15. _____ Snakes can be safely handled just before and during a shed.

16. _____ To help prevent passive reflux of barium into the mouth during a gastrointestinal contrast study, small vet wrap bandage can be placed round the bird's neck close to the mandible.

17. _____ When using a Dremel tool to trim a beak, cover the nares as you hold the beak shut.

18. _____ The general rule of wing trimming is that fewer primary and secondary feathers are removed if the bird is heavier.

19. _____ If a bird is to be microchipped, anesthetize and aseptically prepare the pectoral muscle site.

20. _____ Use greasy or oily medications topically for avian burns.

21. _____ Wood that should not be used for perches includes black locust, oak, and rhododendron.

22. _____ A broken, fully mature, blood feather can lead to the death of a bird.

23. _____ Sweat glands in birds are located at the top of their heads and just below their eyes.

24. _____ Before a shed the skin and eyes of a snake become opaque. Handling should be kept to a minimum at this time.

25. _____ Box turtles have hinged plastrons, so the easiest way to extend their heads is by gently propping open the cranial portion of the carapace and the plastron.

26. _____ Keeping one hand on the neck, just behind the base of skull, will help prevent getting bitten when handling long-necked lizards.

27. _____ All snakes are carnivores and feed on whole prey items.

28. _____ Contrary to popular belief, daily soaking of reptiles will not help improve overall hydration.

29. _____ Urine is not concentrated in the kidneys in birds; rather, urine moves retrograde into the coprodeum and rectum, where resorption of water, sodium, and chloride takes place.

30. _____ Amazon parrots are the only species that will develop hematuria in acute cases of heavy metal toxicosis.

31. _____ Snakes should be offered pre-killed or stunned prey items as food.

32. _____ In order for the cloacal mucosa to be examined properly, it must be everted.

33. _____ Like puppies, birds outgrow the chewing or mouthing stage.

34. _____ Most aquatic turtles are herbivores.

35. _____ Most diseases in exotic animals are caused by poor husbandry and improper diet.

36. _____ When differentiating between genders, male iguanas and bearded dragons have very large femoral pores compared with females.

37. _____ Many species of male tortoises have a concave plastron, making it easier to mount the female.

38. _____ When a snake is being sexed, the probe will advance further into the cloaca of a female snake.

39. _____ EDTA is the anticoagulant used for chemistry evaluation, whereas lithium heparin is the anticoagulant generally used for CBC evaluation in birds and reptiles.

Chapter **12** Avian and Exotic Animal Care and Nursing

40. _____ If a snake is extremely aggressive or if it is a venomous snake, a snake hook should be used to pin down the head of the snake so that its head and body can be safely grasped.

41. _____ Gerbils are permissive hibernators when the temperature is less than 8° C.

42. _____ The anogenital distance is used to differentiate male from female rats, mice, hamsters, and chinchillas.

43. _____ Hamsters can get a vitamin C deficiency if old food is fed to them.

44. _____ Gerbils have a large adrenal gland, increased cholesterol, and lipemic serum.

45. _____ Only the male gerbil has a midventral dark-orange sebaceous gland that is used for territory marking.

46. _____ Hamsters are the species most prone to spontaneous seizures.

47. _____ Chinchillas, like guinea pigs, have open growing teeth, but unlike in guinea pigs dystocia is not common.

48. _____ Ferrets have sweat glands in the skin, and their claws are retractable.

49. _____ It is the sebaceous secretions found in the skin glands that are responsible for the musky odor of ferrets and not the anal glands.

50. _____ Female ferrets are prone to estrogen toxicity with bone marrow suppression and severe anemia if they are not bred once they ovulate.

51. _____ Antibiotics that are generally considered safe for rabbits and rodents are enrofloxacin, chloramphenicol, and ciprofloxacin.

COMPLETE THE CHART

	Genus and Species	Adult Weight (Grams)	Gestation (Days)	Estrous Cycle (Days)	Body Temperature (° C)	Life Span (Years)	Fill in the Blank
Mice						3	Subordinate mice often show evidence of _____
Rat						2½-3½	_____ tumors are quite common
Syrian hamster					38.9		Cheek pouches are _____
Mongolian gerbil	*Meriones unguiculatus*			4-6	37.4-39.0	3	A gerbil is also called a _____
Guinea pig						4–5	Vitamin _____ is a dietary requirement
Chinchilla	*Chinchilla lanigera*			30-50		10	Access to a _____ should be provided as part of the husbandry
Rabbit—New Zealand white				Induced ovulator			Young are called _____
Ferret	*Mustela putorius furo*	0.8-1.2 kg		Induced ovulator		5-8	Susceptible to _____ and should be vaccinated for _____

MULTIPLE CHOICE

1. Which of the following is true with regard to the respiratory system of birds?
    a. Air enters the respiratory system through the nares and continues over an operculum.
    b. An epiglottis is present.
    c. Lobes and alveoli are present so the lungs can inflate.
    d. The diaphragm assists inspiration of air through extension of the intracostal joints.

2. Which of the following is true with regard to air flow in birds?
    a. Birds have a total of five paired air sacs.
    b. The unpaired air sac is the interclavicular air sac.
    c. The respiratory tract cannot communicate with the long bones.
    d. Gas exchange occurs in the air sacs.

3. With regard to the special senses of birds, which statement is not true?
    a. Birds have the traditional five senses: seeing, hearing, feeling, smelling, and tasting.
    b. The vision and hearing control centers are larger than those for taste, touch, and smell.
    c. Bird vision is very acute, and birds can perceive color.
    d. Birds have more taste buds than mammals.

4. Birds bite to:
    a. exhibit dominance.
    b. show affection.
    c. express fear.
    d. both a and c.

5. With the symptoms of disorientation, depression, pneumonia, gastrointestinal upset, kidney and liver damage, or mucous membrane and skin damage in a bird, you might suspect which of the following toxins?
    a. hydrocarbon-based compounds
    b. tobacco
    c. matches
    d. household cleansers

6. Which statement regarding reptilian biology is true?
    a. Like birds, reptiles have a diaphragm to separate the thoracic and abdominal cavities.
    b. There is one visceral cavity, called the *coelom*.
    c. Most reptiles do not have a renal portal system.
    d. Reptile excrement contains two components—urates and feces.

7. Principles of reptilian feeding include which of the following?
    a. Chicken breast, hot dogs, and raw beef provide a complete diet for snakes.
    b. Lizards are usually only herbivorous.
    c. Most aquatic turtles are omnivorous.
    d. Tortoises are omnivores and eat a variety of leaves, grasses, and insects in the wild.

8. With regard to the physical examination, which statement is incorrect?
    a. The kidneys of lizards sit in the pelvic girdle and are palpated via rectal examination.
    b. Septicemia of iguanas is noted as petechiae and ecchymosis on dorsal spines.
    c. Generally, there is a narrow range of normal physiologic values in reptiles.
    d. Heart rates vary depending on temperature, age, species, and health status.

9. An aggressively tight restraint on a bird can result in which of the following?
    a. comfort
    b. respiratory distress
    c. feather loss
    d. death

10. Which of the following is true with regard to examining or restraining amphibians?
   a. It is not necessary to wear nonpowdered vinyl or latex gloves when handling.
   b. The patient should be kept dry when handling to avoid dehydration.
   c. One hand should support the body near the pelvis.
   d. Organs are easily palpated.

11. Which of the following is true with regard to husbandry of reptiles?
   a. The only purpose of cage furniture is to provide a hiding place.
   b. Hot rocks and sizzle stones can cause thermal burns.
   c. Any ultraviolet (UV) lighting will assist reptiles with synthesizing vitamin D.
   d. The green iguana requires decreased levels of humidity to stay healthy.

12. Which of the following is true with regard to amphibian care and feeding?
   a. Temperature, pH, salinity, and hardness of water should be checked on a regular basis.
   b. Nitrogenous waste buildup and disinfectant residues are easily tolerated.
   c. Alkalinity, dissolved oxygen, and nitrate need not be checked on a regular basis.
   d. Most amphibians are herbivores as adults.

13. Which of the following is true with regard to performing a venipuncture of amphibians?
   a. Alcohol is best used to clean the venipuncture site.
   b. Venipuncture in salamanders is generally performed using the caudal tail vein.
   c. A 20- to 22-gauge needle attached to a 1.0-mL syringe should be used.
   d. The femoral and lingual veins are commonly used in frogs and toads, whereas the ventral abdominal vein is the most difficult to use.

14. Feather mutilation and plucking are common behaviors of which bird species?
   a. cockatoos
   b. pigeons
   c. canaries
   d. parrots

15. The fecal slide you are examining shows gram-positive bacterial flora and some yeast. You are likely examining the feces of which bird grouping?
   a. raptors
   b. galliforms
   c. grain- and fruit-eating psittaciforms
   d. anseriformes

MATCHING

1. _____ Squamata		A. Turtles, tortoises
2. _____ Anura		B. Salamanders
3. _____ Testudines		C. Rodents
4. _____ Caudata		D. Snakes, lizards
5. _____ Gymnophiona		E. Rodents
6. _____ Chelonian		F. Frogs, toads
7. _____ Muridae		G. Caecilians
8. _____ Lagomorphs		H. Rabbits

Define the terms.

1. Pneumatic: _____

2. Synsacrum: _____

3. Operculum: _____

4. Coprodeum: _____

5. Diurnal: _____

6. Malocclusion: _____

7. Coprophagic: _____

8. Jill: _____

9. Rodent: _____

10. Barbering: _____

11. Anisodactyl: _____

12. Apteria: _____

PHOTO QUIZ

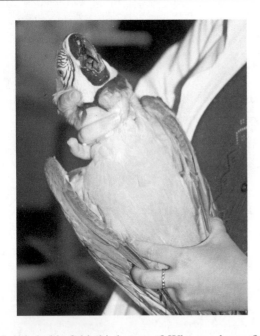

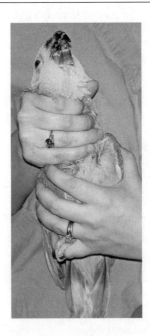

1. Is this hold of this bird correct? Why or why not?

   _____

   _____

2. Is this the correct restraint for this parrot? Why or why not?

   _____

   _____

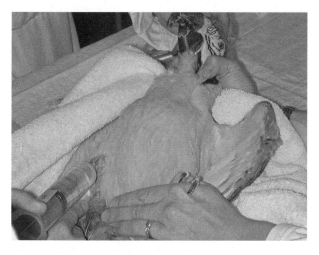

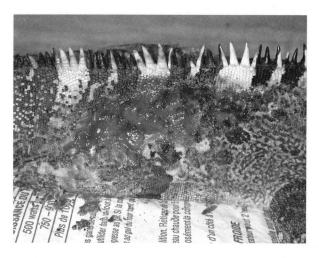

3. The site for these subcutaneous fluids is _____; this is the site of choice because _____. Use a _____ -gauge needle.

4. What is the likely cause of this condition?

_____

_____

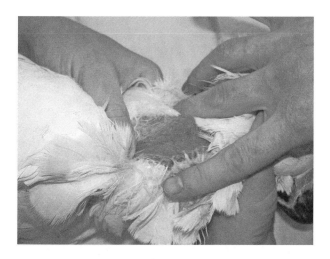

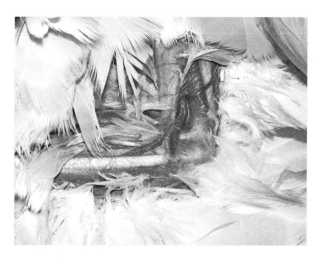

5. Is this site appropriate for a small bird?

_____

_____

6. Why should the _____ not be used routinely for blood collection?

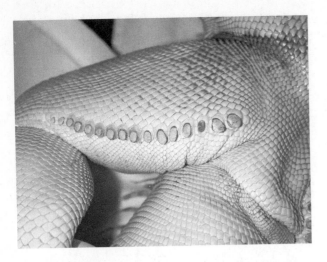

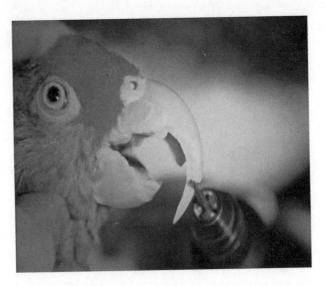

7. Are the femoral pores shown characteristic of male or female lizards?

_____

_____

8. The instrument used to trim this beak is a _____.

Do not cover the _____ when restraining the beak.

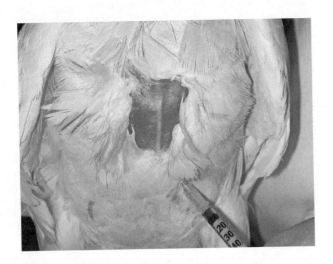

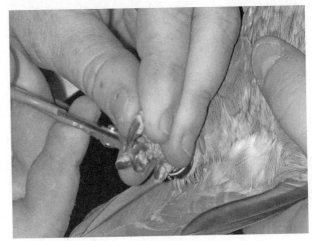

9. Use no more than _____ mL in a large bird in this IM site.

10. Why are regular nail trims important?

_____

_____

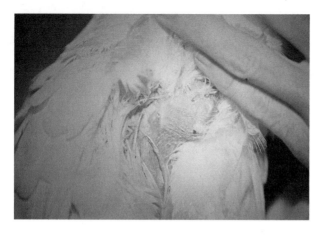

11. The cause of crop fistula in this hand-fed juvenile cockatoo is likely _____

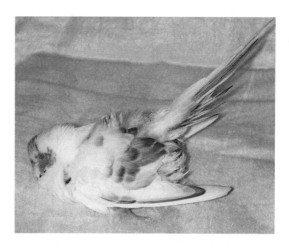

12. This bird is showing signs of _____.

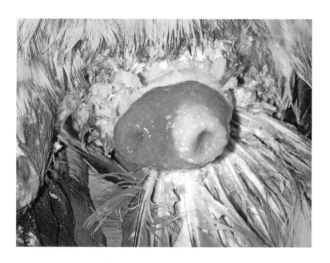

13. The most important immediate therapy for a prolapsed cloaca is to _____.

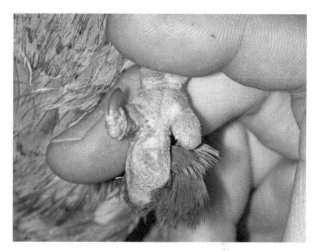

14. Name the condition being exhibited by this bird.

_____

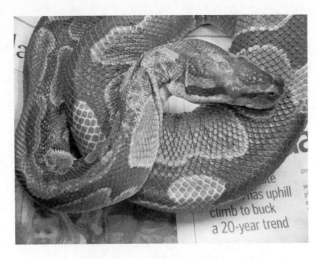

15. This snake's skin and eyes are turning an opaque blue color. What is happening?

_____

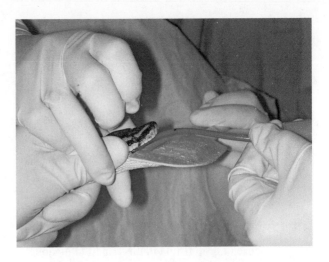

16. What procedure is being completed in this picture? Is the device used the correct one?

_____

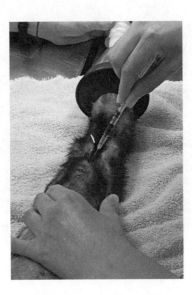

17. Name the blood vessel being used for blood collection.

_____

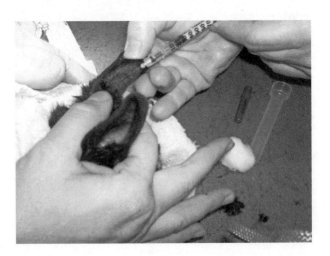

18. Name the blood vessel being used for blood collection.

_____

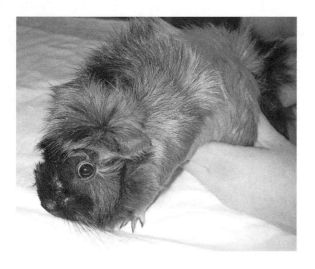

19. Name this breed of guinea pig.

_____

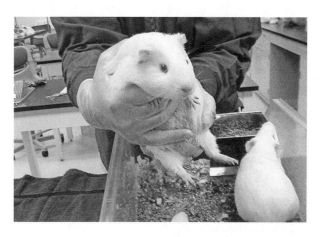

20. Is this a correct method for removal of this species from a cage? Why or why not?

_____

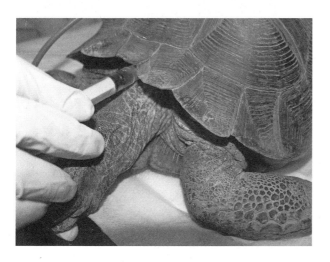

21. What site is being used, and how is the blood obtained?

_____

_____

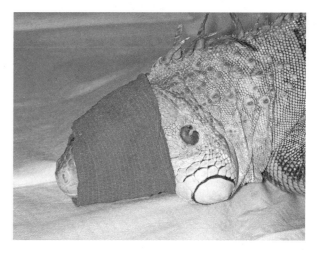

22. What is the purpose of the cotton balls over the eye and an elastic wrap?

_____

_____

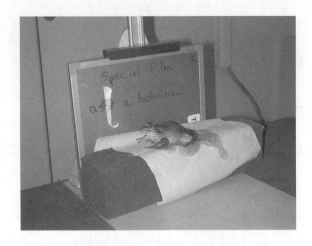

23. What view is being taken?

_____

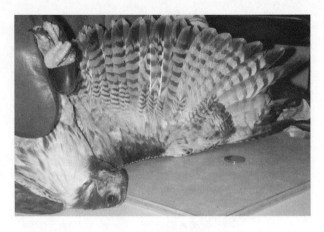

24. What view is being prepared?

_____

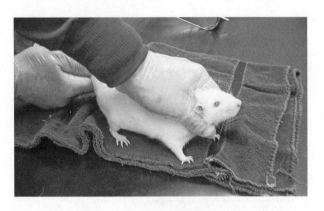

25. Is this correct restraint for this rodent? Why or why not?

_____

_____

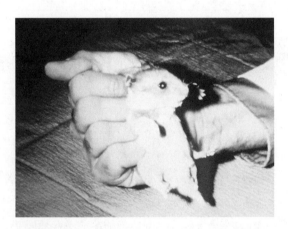

26. Is this the proper hold for an intraperitoneal injection? Why or why not?

_____

_____

CROSSWORD

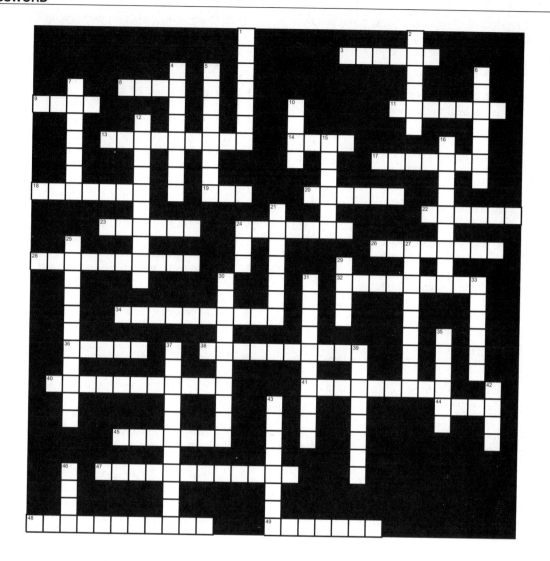

Chapter **12** Avian and Exotic Animal Care and Nursing

Across

3 The end product of nitrogenous waste production from the liver that is excreted by the kidney as a pasty white to yellow material found in bird droppings

8 A female ferret

9 The dilatation of the esophagus located at the base of the neck just cranial to the thoracic inlet

11 Contour feathers found on the wing of a bird; the flight feathers

13 When a dominant mouse chews the fur of a subordinate mouse

14 A male rabbit

17 The featherless areas of birds where there are no feather tracts

18 Nine thin, transparent membranes that are connected to the primary and secondary bronchi and act as reservoirs for air entering and leaving the lungs

19 A female guinea pig

20 Feeding with a tube passed through the oral cavity into the stomach

22 The voice box of birds

23 The body cavity in birds that extends from the first thoracic rib to the vent

24 Pertaining to those species that forage or hunt in the daytime

26 A surveillance animal housed for the purpose of identifying abnormal occurrences

28 Perching birds and songbirds such as canaries, finches, and sparrows

32 A keratinized flap of tissue inside the nares of some birds

34 Gnawing mammals that have two pairs or incisors in the upper jaw, one behind the other

36 A common name for guinea pigs

38 The caudal part of the cloaca that empties contents into the vent

40 Filled with air

41 The middle ear bone in birds

44 The fleshy colored skin located at the base of the upper beak in many bird species

45 The middle compartment of the cloaca that is terminal end to the ureters and genital ducts

47 Improper positioning of teeth

48 Gizzard

49 Smaller feathers that cover the remiges and rectrices

Down

1 The process of feather replacement that occurs one to several times a year, depending on the species

2 A dark ribbonlike structure attached to the retina and extending into the vitreous humor and thought to provide nourishment to the eye

4 Loss of hair

5 Itching

6 Feather tracts on the skin of birds

7 The __ feathers are the largest feathers that form the external appearance of adult birds

10 Male ferrets

15 The V-shaped notch in the roof of the mouth of birds that provides communication between the nasal cavity and the oropharynx

16 The __ gland secretes a lipoid sebaceous material that is spread over feathers during preening to help with waterproofing

21 Also known as *pododermatitis*: an inflammation of the ball of the foot of birds and guinea pigs

24 A female rabbit

25 Parrots, macaws, and parakeets

27 Pertaining to species that forage and hunt at night

29 A male guinea pig

30 The terminal end of the rectum in the cranial compartment of the cloaca

31 The feet of psittacines that are shaped so that the second and third toes point forward and the first and fourth toes are directed backward

33 Pertaining to mice or rats

35 The terminal end for the reproductive, urinary, and gastrointestinal tracts

37 The foot of passerines with three toes that point forward and one toe that points to the rear

39 A term used to describe a juvenile parrot using the tongue to explore surfaces

42 The bony ridge on the sternum of birds where the flight muscles attach

43 Capable of being transmitted from animals to human beings

46 The __ is a layer of fine feathers under the exterior feathers

13 Large Animal Nursing and Husbandry

LEARNING OBJECTIVES

After reviewing this chapter, the reader will be able to:

- Describe the general husbandry needs of large animals.
- Describe restraint methods used with large animals.
- Explain and demonstrate routine procedures used in grooming and foot care.
- Discuss the techniques used in general nursing care of large animals.
- Discuss the methods of sample collection for laboratory analysis.
- Compare and contrast various routes of administration of medication in large animals.
- Identify and describe various methods of sample collection for laboratory analysis.

FILL IN THE BLANK

1. A _____ is any dietary component that provides some essential nutrient or serves some other function.

2. _____ are feeds made up of most or all of the plant.

3. _____ is the most common grain fed to livestock.

4. Because calves are born essentially _____, provision of colostrum shortly after birth is critically important.

5. For calves with fluid loss because of neonatal enteritis, _____ solutions are commonly offered as a means to provide additional fluid therapy.

6. Silage is not commonly fed to horses because of their sensitivity to the _____ and _____ potentially found in silage.

7. _____ produces less dust and may be better for horses recovering from respiratory allergies or pneumonia.

8. Pig diets consist primarily of _____, along with energy, protein, mineral, and vitamin supplements.

9. Goats may be used for _____, _____, or _____ production.

10. Physical assessment of production animals may include observations of hair coat, _____, hydration status, manure consistency, and attitude.

11. Black walnut shavings can cause _____ when the horse stands in the shavings.

12. Topical fly sprays that contain _____, _____, or _____ are safest for sick horses.

13. The horse's hoof is cleaned with a hoof pick by removing debris from the lateral and central sulci, starting at the _____ and working toward the _____, and then from the rest of the hoof.

14. The intact adult male swine is a _____, and the castrated male is called a _____.

15. An alert horse has its ears _____.

1. _____ Fly repellents containing organophosphates should not be applied to debilitated horses or foals.

2. _____ A body condition score of 1 represents an emaciated animal.

3. _____ Pigs are omnivores.

4. _____ A metal curry comb should be used in a circular motion to remove dried sweat or mud from the horse's face.

5. _____ A degenerative condition called *thrush* is common in feet that are infrequently cleaned.

6. _____ A castrated male sheep is called a *ram*.

7. _____ Young female swine are called *gilts* until they farrow.

8. _____ An angry or fearful horse often pins its ears forward.

9. _____ Horses should be approached from the front and slightly to the near (left) side.

10. _____ Always stand on the opposite side of the horse as the person who is working on the animal.

MATCHING

Select the proper male or female name for the following animals.

1. _____ Adult intact male ovine

2. _____ Male adult bovine

3. _____ Adult female porcine

4. _____ Young female porcine before farrowing

5. _____ Adult female ovine

6. _____ Adult intact male caprine

7. _____ Castrated male porcine

8. _____ Female adult bovine

9. _____ Castrated male ovines/caprines

10. _____ Adult female caprine

11. _____ Male castrated bovine

12. _____ Young ovine

13. _____ Female young adult bovine

14. _____ Young porcine

15. _____ Intact adult male porcine

A. Gilt

B. Bull

C. Piglet

D. Doe

E. Lamb

F. Sow

G. Heifer

H. Buck/Ram

I. Boar

J. Cow

K. Wether

L. Billy/Ram

M. Steer

N. Ewe

O. Barrow

Match the breed name to the image on the left.

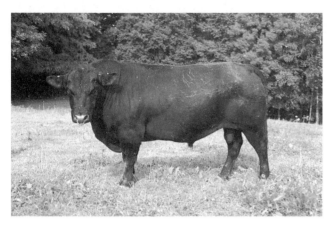

A. Holstein

1. (From Sambraus HH: A colour atlas of livestock breeds. London, Mosby-Wolfe, 1992.)

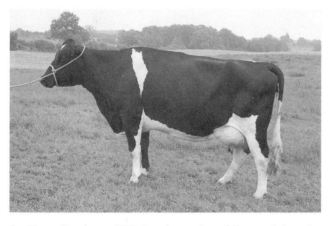

B. Texas Longhorn

2. (From Sambraus HH: A colour atlas of livestock breeds. London, Mosby-Wolfe, 1992.)

C. Angus

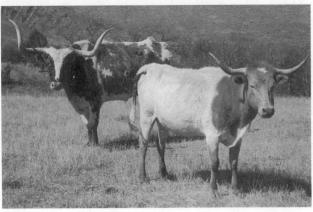

3. (From Sambraus HH: A colour atlas of livestock breeds. London, Mosby-Wolfe, 1992.)

D. Hereford

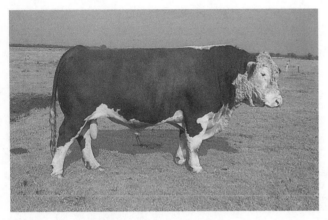

4. (From Sambraus HH: A colour atlas of livestock breeds. London, Mosby-Wolfe, 1992.)

WORD SEARCH

```
T  G  N  I  W  O  R  R  A  F  C  M  C  A  I
H  B  N  O  J  K  L  B  M  D  K  O  M  A  L
R  C  E  I  I  A  T  M  M  X  L  E  T  R  N
U  G  O  Y  A  T  T  S  A  O  T  K  C  P  W
S  S  I  G  V  H  A  K  S  S  I  L  T  F  J
H  H  I  T  C  W  C  T  A  M  V  S  P  L  E
B  K  Q  L  E  Q  R  I  S  M  T  I  A  S  B
V  P  R  T  A  O  D  H  F  E  Q  T  L  Q  N
Y  C  H  E  M  G  Q  T  O  L  G  I  Y  Q  P
Q  E  Z  E  X  V  E  Y  E  B  L  N  G  A  M
R  S  T  S  U  L  O  B  Z  G  O  I  B  G  R
Y  E  F  F  T  Y  Q  V  U  N  E  M  P  G  A
R  T  W  I  T  C  H  H  V  J  R  A  V  Y  W
Y  X  E  D  M  I  J  Q  X  O  H  L  G  H  C
V  G  N  V  U  L  D  Q  Q  J  I  M  T  M  G
```

BOLUS	CHAIN	COLOSTROMETER
DIASTEMA	FARROWING	GESTATION
LAMINITIS	SILAGE	THRUSH
TWITCH	WETHER	

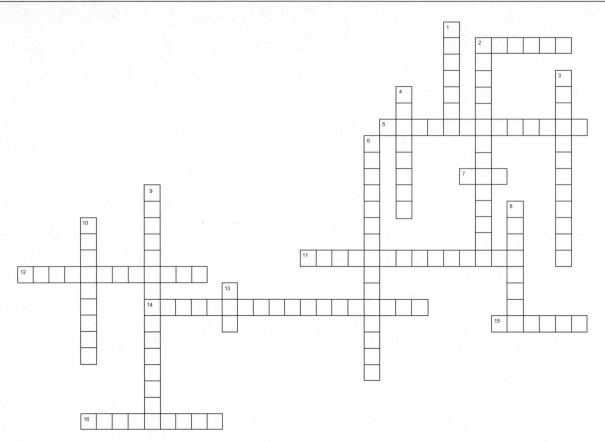

Across

2 Castrated male sheep
5 Tool that measures the specific gravity of the colostrum
7 Intact adult male sheep
11 Residues of the feed-processing industry
12 Metal clamplike device that pinches the upper lip between two bars
14 Without immunoglobulins
15 Castrated male pig
16 Any dietary component that provides some essential nutrient or serves some other function

Down

1 Used on dairy cattle that have tendency to kick the milkers
2 Minimum length of time that must pass from the last administration of the medicine until the time that the animal is slaughtered for food or the milk
3 Restraint device used almost exclusively on beef cattle
4 Forage harvested at a given stage of development and fed directly
6 Pregnancy length
8 Pressure sores
9 Interdental space
10 Giving small volumes of liquids po
13 Forage that is cut and allowed to dry before being collected into bales for storage